Arnould-Tay

Principles and Practice o|

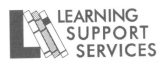

Physical

Stanley Thornes (Publishers) Ltd

First published in 1977 for
Arnould-Taylor Education Ltd
2nd Edition 1982
3rd Edition 1991
4th Edition 1997

by
Stanley Thornes (Publishers) Ltd
Ellenborough House
Wellington Street
Cheltenham GL50 1YW
UK

98 99 00 01 / 10 9 8 7 6 5 4 3 2

A catalogue record for this book is available from the British Library.

ISBN 0-7487-2998-4

Companion volumes to this title

A TEXTBOOK OF HOLISTIC AROMATHERAPY by W. Arnould-Taylor

A TEXTBOOK OF ANATOMY AND PHYSIOLOGY by W. Arnould-Taylor

PRINCIPLES AND PRACTICE OF PERFUMERY AND COSMETICS
by G. Howard and W. Arnould-Taylor

Typeset by Florencetype Ltd, Stoodleigh, Devon

Printed and bound in Italy
by G. Canale & C. S.p.A. – Borgaro T.se – Turin

Contents

Preface to the 4th Edition

Over the years since the first edition of this book in 1977, I have added to the text as new information has become available. Now, in consultation with the publishers, it has been decided to broaden the scope of the book.

For the new chapters I invited contributions from experts in their respective fields. I hope readers will agree that this additional knowledge, together with the general up-dating of the original text, combines to increase the value of the book as a whole.

I would like to record my appreciation of the contributions by Paul Godwin, Sean Blake, John Beney and Jane Evans, and also of the continuous help, suggestions and guidance of my colleague Kim Aldridge, and of Neal Marriott, Louise Watson and Stephanie Richards at Stanley Thornes.

My thanks also go to Amanda Cornford for granting permission to reproduce her poem *The Skeleton in Rhyme* on pages 24–5.

William Arnould-Taylor
Oxford, 1997

The Study of Anatomy and Physiology

A review of standard textbooks on anatomy and physiology reveals that the majority are written with the medical student or nurse particularly in mind and few, if any, have been written specifically for the physical therapist. The result is that the physical therapist often has to wade through a good deal of material which is going to be largely valueless to him or her in the practice of the profession. The difference of approach between, say, a nurse on the one hand and a physical therapist on the other, is a basic one – the nurse is primarily concerned with what happens *inside* the body, that is beneath the skin, whereas the physical therapist is more concerned with the *exterior* of the body and those parts of the body which may be influenced from the exterior.

It has been found that very detailed textbooks on anatomy and physiology, though excellent for medical and nursing students, leave other students a little confused as to what is most suitable for them to select for the purposes of their studies. It is hoped, therefore, that this comparatively small section on anatomy and physiology will help to fill the gap. It makes no pretence of enveloping the whole of the subject matter of anatomy and physiology but aims to provide a basic understanding of the relative parts of the body and their functions.

1 Introduction to Anatomy and Physiology

It is important to have a clear understanding of the difference between the two terms – anatomy and physiology. Anatomy is normally defined as being the study of the *structure* of the body and the relationship of various parts one to another; whereas physiology is the study of the *functions* of those parts. For example, to say that the human heart is approximately 255 g in weight, is somewhat pear-shaped in appearance and lies two-thirds to the left-hand side of the rib cage and one-third to the right, is to describe its anatomy; that is its weight, shape and position. On the other hand, this information tells us nothing at all about the function of the heart so we have to look at the physiology to learn that the heart is basically a pump which forces oxygenated blood around the body and, at the same time, circulates the venous or carbon dioxide loaded blood around the lungs for reoxygenisation.

Therefore, by combining the knowledge of anatomy and physiology of the heart we are able to get a picture of what it looks like as well as what it does. In the ensuing chapters anatomy and physiology are dealt with together.

For the purpose of simplicity of learning, the body is divided into eight systems. In some textbooks these basic systems are sub-divided so that nine, ten or more systems are quoted. However, on closer investigation, it will be seen that these additional systems are really part of the basic systems. These we divide as follows:

- the *skeletal system* which, as its name implies, is the bony structure on which the other systems depend for support
- the *muscular system*
- the *vascular system* which includes the lymphatic system
- the *neurological system* which covers all the nerves of the body as well as the brain.

3

These four systems we refer to as the *major systems*, not because they are more important than the systems which follow, but because they are the systems which envelop the whole of the body and are the ones which can most easily be affected by the professional skills of the physical therapist.

We now pass on to:

- the *digestive system*
- the *respiratory system*
- the *genito-urinary system* which includes the reproductive and kidney systems
- the *endocrine system*.

These last four systems are referred to as the *minor systems*.

All professions have their own peculiar vocabularies – these are necessary for the accurate understanding of the subject matter – and the profession of medicine is no exception. It has a very wide vocabulary which requires a lifetime to master fully. There are, however, parts of this vocabulary which are essential to the physical therapist and these are dealt with in the form of a glossary at the end of each chapter so as not to interfere with the flow of the text of the lesson itself. It is important that you try to understand this terminology, because, if the words are learnt in relation to the appropriate discussion, it makes the subsequent learning that much easier.

A *brief history*

It is not possible to trace the beginnings of the study of anatomy and physiology for these are lost in antiquity. The ancient Egyptians were famous for their embalming processes which must have involved a certain amount of knowledge of the anatomy of the human body and they had a system of medicine, traces of which survive until today. The R which a doctor writes at the top of his prescription is, in fact, the 'R' symbol for the Eye of Horus – the hawk-headed sun god who lost his eye in battle and had it restored by Thoth, the patron god of physicians. Thoth was one of the many gods invoked by doctors of ancient Egypt when administering their remedies.

About the same time, but in an entirely different part of the world, the Chinese were practising a form of medicine, acupuncture, which involved some 365 different needling points, but it is to the civilisation of the Greek period that we have to look for more detailed knowledge of human anatomy.

From this era we have the work of Hippocrates, who is often referred to as the father of medicine, and, in a rather different role, the name of Aristotle, who is generally acknowledged as being the founder of comparative anatomy.

During the Roman period which followed there was a medical school in Rome, and the fine selection of surgical and dissecting instruments which have been preserved indicates a considerable knowledge of the structure of the human body.

Galen lived in the second century and his name is still remembered as being that of one of the greatest physicians and anatomists of antiquity. His work formed the basis of the European knowledge of anatomy for well over a thousand years, surviving through the Dark Ages into the Middle Ages when we see the beginning of the great Italian medical schools and universities such as Bologna and Padua. One of the sixteenth-century graduates was Paracelsus von Hohenheim, a progressive medical teacher, who did much to alter the accepted ideas of his day. It was in 1543 that Versalius published his first drawings of the structure of the human body and so paved the way for modern anatomy. Nearly a hundred years later, in 1628, Harvey announced his discovery of the role of the heart in the circulation of the blood through the lungs and the body, and in 1661 Malpighi discovered the capillary circulation and so completed the knowledge of how blood from arteries is returned to the heart by way of veins.

In the middle of the eighteenth century Auenbrugger of Austria invented percussion – a method by which doctors could diagnose the condition of the lungs. As a boy he had often watched his father tap barrels to see how much wine they contained and he applied the same technique to the chests of his patients. If they gave out hollow sounds similar to those of empty barrels he considered they were healthy, whilst a muffled or high-pitched note indicated the presence of some unhealthy fluid.

At the end of the eighteenth century – 1798 – Jenner discovered that vaccination could be employed as a preventive of smallpox. Early in the nineteenth century the French physician, Rene Laennec, invented the stethoscope. He was attending a patient suffering from heart disease and, as she was rather obese, he decided that applying an ear direct to the chest (which was the usual method) would be of little use. He remembered that children sometimes amused themselves by playing with logs of wood, one child making tapping or scratching noises at one end and the other one listening at the other. So he rolled up a cylinder of paper and put one end of the stethoscope to the patient's chest and his ear to the other and found that he could hear the heart beating much more clearly than before. He then experimented with other materials until the stethoscope was invented.

The first real knowledge of the digestive system came in 1822 when a man by the name of Alexis St Martin was wounded in the stomach during a brawl near Lake Michigan. He recovered but the wound left a permanent hole through which Dr William Beaumont, US Army, was able to watch how the stomach exuded the juices needed for digestion.

In the 1840s nitrous oxide or laughing gas was first used by a dentist in America for the extraction of teeth. This was quickly followed by the use of ether in hospital operating theatres which made possible a much more detailed study of anatomy. In 1867 Lister established the principles of antisepsis and in 1877 Pasteur demonstrated the role of germs in the causation of disease. In 1895 Röntgen discovered X-rays and in 1898 the Curies isolated radium. In 1904 Bayliss and Starling identified the first hormone. The year 1912 saw the discovery of vitamins by Frederick Gowland Hopkins, whilst in 1928 Alexander

Fleming discovered the antibiotic – penicillin – though this was not to come into medical use until about 1939.

Anatomy and physiology are subjects of continuous research and discovery and all the knowledge which has accumulated in this century serves to indicate that we are only at the beginning of a complete understanding of these two subjects.

GLOSSARY

Some general terms used in anatomy and physiology.

Acute	sharp, severe; of short duration
The anatomical position	an erect position of the human body with arms by sides and palms of the hands facing forward
Anterior	applies to the front of the body when in the erect position
Chronic	of long duration
Distal	the opposite of proximal and the part furthest away from the median line; so distal thigh will be at the knee end of the thigh
Dorsal	synonymous with posterior; normally used when describing the hand or the foot
Hydro	fluid
Hyper	above, in excess of normal
Hypo	below, less than normal
Itis	inflammation
Lateral	either side of the median line, e.g. the outer side of the arm will be its lateral aspect whilst the inner side is described as the medial aspect
Median line	an imaginary line which runs through the centre of the body from the centre of the crown of the head ending up directly between the two feet
Morphology	the study of differences and resemblances in structure and form
Posterior	the back of the body when in the erect position
Proximal	a term of comparison applied to structures which are nearer the centre of the body or the median line, e.g. proximal thigh is the end of the thigh nearest to the centre of the body
Psuedo	false
Symmetrical	similar parts of the body, e.g. right and left ears, eyes, tibias, or limbs

2 Histology

Histology can be readily defined in two words – *microscopic anatomy*. It is the branch of biology which deals with the minute structure of tissues which are the basis of cell life.

Cells

All living structures are composed of cells and intercellular material. Some of this intercellular material provides strength, for example, collagen and elastic fibres in the skin and calcium salts in the bone, whilst much of the intercellular material acts as a cement between the cells. This is sometimes referred to a *ground substance* or *interstitial substance*.

Life starts when a single ovum (female sex cell) is fertilised by a spermatozoon (male sex cell). These sex cells are formed by a process, meiosis, in which the number of *chromosomes* (genetic material) in the nucleus is halved.

This fertilised cell consists of a nucleus, containing the full complement of chromosomes, surrounded by protoplasm and enclosed by a membrane. It divides by a process called *mitosis*, in which the essential elements of the nucleus, the chromosomes, are reproduced in each daughter cell. The chromosomes are made up of a linear arrangement of genes. It is now known that the genes in each cell (*genome*) contain a complete pattern of the human body.

In 1943 it was discovered that genes were made from very long, large molecules of *deoxyribonucleic acid*, DNA for short, but the way in which DNA carried all the information to produce a complete human being remained unknown until 1953. It was then discovered that DNA was made of four different small molecules called *nucleotides* linked together in a long chain. The most important feature of DNA is that two of these very long chains twist around each other to form a double helix rather like a rubber ladder twisted around its long axis. The DNA molecule is by far the largest molecule found in the cell, which is not surprising, considering the amount of information it has to carry in its four letter alphabet.

In each cell there are something like 30 000 million such letters, equivalent to 1000 books of 1000 pages each. It will be seen that the genes carry the determining factors of inheritance and cell behaviour.

Gradually, as a result of mitosis, a ball of cells is formed and in the very early stages this ball of cells can be divided into three layers:

- an outer layer – the *ectoderm* or *epiblast* from which the skin, its appendages and the nervous system are developed
- a middle layer – the *mesoderm* or *mesoblast* from which fat and various internal organs are developed
- an inner layer – the *endoblast* which provides the lining of a number of organs of the body.

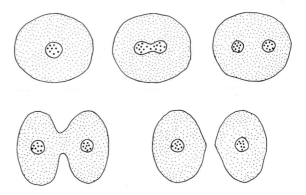

CELL MITOSIS

So the single cell has developed into tissue and, when fully developed, there are four types of tissue in the body:

- *the epithelium*
- *connective tissue*
- *muscular tissue*
- *nerve tissue.*

Epithelium

The epithelium is divided into two principal types:

- *simple epithelium* which consists of one layer of cells. It is very delicate and is found in several organ linings like the thorax and the abdomen
- *stratified* or *compound epithelium* which consists of two or more layers.

Connective tissue

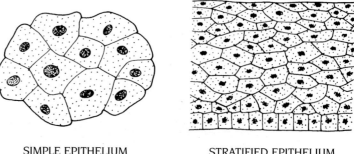

SIMPLE EPITHELIUM   STRATIFIED EPITHELIUM

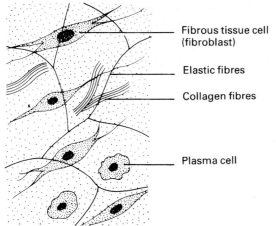

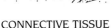

Fibrous tissue cell (fibroblast)

Elastic fibres

Collagen fibres

Plasma cell

CONNECTIVE TISSUE

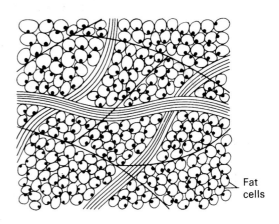

Fat cells

FAT CELLS BOUNDED BY WHITE CONNECTIVE TISSUE FIBRES

This connects all other tissues and, when presented in the form of bone, gives support and rigidity to the body. There are seven principal types of connective tissue:

- *areolar* or *loose connective tissue*, which forms a very thin transparent tissue which surrounds vessels, nerves and muscle fibres
- *adipose tissue*, which is not unlike loose connective tissue but the spaces of the network are filled in with fat cells
- *fibrous tissue*, which is found in tendons and ligaments and also forms the outside of various organs such as the kidney and heart, as well as the outside of bone and muscle
- *bone*, which is a special type of fibrous material hardened by the deposit of such salts as calcium phosphate, the fibrous material giving it toughness and the mineral matter giving it rigidity
- *cartilage*, which is a specialised type of fibrous tissue. It is tough and pliable and very strong. It provides a firm wall to the larynx and the trachea and for the pads which join bone to bone in the slightly movable joints, for example between the vertebrae
- *yellow elastic tissue*, which is found where elasticity is important as in the walls of blood vessels

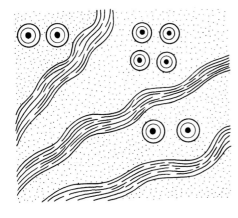

WHITE FIBROCARTILAGE

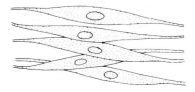

SMOOTH MUSCLE FIBRE

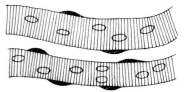

STRIATED MUSCLE FIBRE

- *lymphoid or reticular tissue*, which is found in lymph nodes and the spleen.

Muscular tissue

Muscular tissue is contractile tissue and is able to produce movement. This is dealt with in more detail in Chapter 4, The Muscular System.

Nerve tissue

Nerve tissue has the special function of carrying messages or stimuli throughout the body. It consists of nerve cells and nerve fibres and is dealt with in greater detail in Chapter 6, The Neurological System.

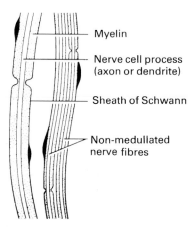

Myelin

Nerve cell process (axon or dendrite)

Sheath of Schwann

Non-medullated nerve fibres

NERVE TISSUE

In addition to the tissues mentioned above, there are three liquid or fluid tissues – the *blood*, *lymph* and *cerebro-spinal fluid* (see Chapters 5 and 6).

Membranes

Membranes are made of connective tissue and line the cavities and hollow organs of the body. They secrete lubricating fluids to moisten their smooth surfaces and prevent friction. There are three types of membrane found in the human body:

- *synovial membrane*, which secretes a very thick fluid rather like egg white in consistency
- *mucous membrane*, which secretes a sticky fluid called *mucus*
- *serous membrane*, which is made of flattened cells through which a small quantity of a thin, watery substance oozes. The fluid which emanates from it is called *serum*.

Waterlogging of the tissues can occur and when this happens it is called *oedema*. This can arise from a number of causes:

- too high hydrostatic pressure in the capillaries
- an osmotic pressure that is too low
- a blockage of lymphatic vessels
- damage to the capillary walls.

Cardiac oedema occurs in congestive heart trouble and this is caused by the increase in venous pressure and the consequent increase in capillary pressure. It is characterised by swelling of the legs and feet of those who habitually walk or stand, whilst it appears in the lower part of the back or buttocks of those who lie. An important factor is the kidneys and their diminished secretion of sodium.

Summary

Human beings start as a single cell formed by the fusion of two sex cells. Mitosis is the process by which a cell multiplies.

Most tissues are dealt with under their respective headings but this chapter has primarily been concerned with connective tissue which serves as the supporting system of the body. Its cells are responsible for the elements and matrix of bone, cartilaginous and fibrous tissue. They form the various tough frameworks of the body, whilst the matrix supplies lubricating elements which facilitate easy movement.

Collagen was, at one time, used synonymously with connective tissue but is now used more specifically to indicate connective tissue fibres.

Ground substance is a type of cementing material found between the minute fibres, binding them together.

HIV

HIV (*human immuno deficiency virus*) is a retrovirus which is different from other viruses in that its genetic message is stored in a molecule called RNA (ribonucleic acid). Other viruses have their genetic messages stored in DNA. In retroviruses the message goes in the reverse direction, which makes it harder to eradicate.

HIV attacks and fights the cells of the immune system. A molecule named CP120 can bind itself to a molecule called CD4 in the cell walls of helper T lymphocytes. These T cells are the principal kind of cell depleted in the course of HIV disease. Once HIV has inserted its message, it is there for the life of the cell and can only be eliminated if the cell is killed.

HIV can remain in a dormant state for as long as 12 years, although it is most infectious during the first three months. Once it is activated (usually by certain other infections), the viral DNA is converted into viral RNA using enzymes to make viral proteins. The various viral proteins migrate to the surface of the T cells and are assembled there. These new viruses are emitted from the cell wall and go on to infect other cells.

Although HIV has been isolated from several body fluids, the only means of transmission that are documented by research are by way of blood, semen, vaginal secretions, contaminated hypodermic needles, mother to child during pregnancy and birth, and organ transplants.

In common with other viruses, HIV has the ability to transmute (the influenza virus is a good example), so we may see changes in the development and treatment of this disease.

GLOSSARY

Centrosome	a very small dense part of the cytoplasm lying close to the nucleus
Chromosomes	thread-shaped bodies consisting of DNA, found in the nucleus of the cell. There are 23 pairs (46 in total) in each human cell
Genes	hereditary determinants occurring in the chromosomes in linear arrangement
Grand cytoplasm	a type of protoplasm surrounding the nucleus, in which the other structures are embedded
Golgi apparatus	a canal-like structure lying close to the nucleus; named after the famous Italian histologist who first described it at the beginning of the twentieth century
Karyokinesis	same as mitosis – cell division
Meiosis	the type of cell division which takes place in the sex organs. The number of chromosomes is halved so that a spermatazoon provides 23 chromosomes and the ovum 23 chromosomes
Mitochondria	small, rodlike structures embedded in the cytoplasm
Pathology	a branch of science which deals with the nature of disease through the study of cause, process, effect and associated alternations of structure and function

3 The Skeletal System

The skeleton provides the framework of the body and it has two principal functions. The first is that of *protection*, for example:

- **the skull protects the brain**
- **the rib cage protects principally the heart and the lungs**
- **the spinal column protects the spinal cord**
- **the pelvic bones provide a certain amount of protection for the viscera.**

The second function is that of *locomotion*, or *movement*.

Bones

The skeleton is made up of 206 *bones*, though this figure varies slightly in different textbooks due to the fact that some authorities count the number of bones which are present in a young child, whereas other authorities consider that only the bones of an adult should be counted, as by the time adulthood is reached certain childhood bones will have fused together.

Bone is a dry dense tissue composed of approximately 25 per cent water, 30 per cent organic material and 45 per cent mineral. The mineral matter consists chiefly of calcium phosphate and a small amount of magnesium salts; these give the bone its rigidity and hardness. The organic matter consists of fibrous material which gives the bone its toughness and resilience. There are five classifications of bone:

- *long bones*, e.g. the femur or thigh bone, the longest and strongest bone of the body
- *short bones*, e.g. tarsal bones
- *flat bones*, e.g. frontal bone of the head
- *irregular bones*, e.g. the vertebrae
- *sesamoid bones*, which are rounded masses found in certain tendons of muscles, the best example being the patella or knee cap.

A long bone normally consists of marrow surrounded by a spongy bone layer which, in turn, is surrounded by a compact bone layer and finally by a hard outside covering known as the periosteum.

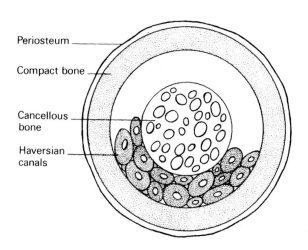

Periosteum

Compact bone

Cancellous bone

Haversian canals

A SECTION THROUGH
A LONG BONE

In addition to the two principal functions of the skeleton, individual bones serve other purposes such as the attachment of tendons and muscles, and the formation of red blood cells and some white blood cells in the bone marrow.

Joints

A *joint* is formed where two bones meet. Joints may be divided according to their mobility, into three types:

- fixed joints
- slightly movable joints
- freely movable joints.

Fixed joints

Fixed joints, or *synarthroses*, provide no movement, for example the sutures between the skull bones. There is fibrous tissue between the bones, which either overlap or are fitted together in a jagged line.

Slightly movable joints

Slightly movable joints, or *amphiathroses*, are found in the pelvis (*symphysis pubis*), sacro-iliac joint and the joints at both ends of the clavicle. The bones are held together by strong ligaments and separated by pads of fibrocartilage (*cartilaginous joints*).

Freely movable joints

Freely movable joints are enclosed in a fibrous capsule, supported by ligaments. This capsule is lined by a *synovial membrane* with *synovial fluid* in the cavity. This is a whitish fluid, not unlike raw egg-white in consistency, which acts like oil in a machine to reduce friction between the articulating surfaces of the joint. The bone surfaces are covered by *hyaline cartilage* for smoother operation.

There are four main groups of freely movable joints:

- *ball and socket articulations* – hip joint, shoulder joint
- *hinge articulations* – knee joint (full hinge), elbow joint (partial hinge)
- *pivot articulations* – radius and ulna joints, axis joint of cervical spine
- *gliding joints* – tarsal joint of ankle, carpal joint of wrist.

14

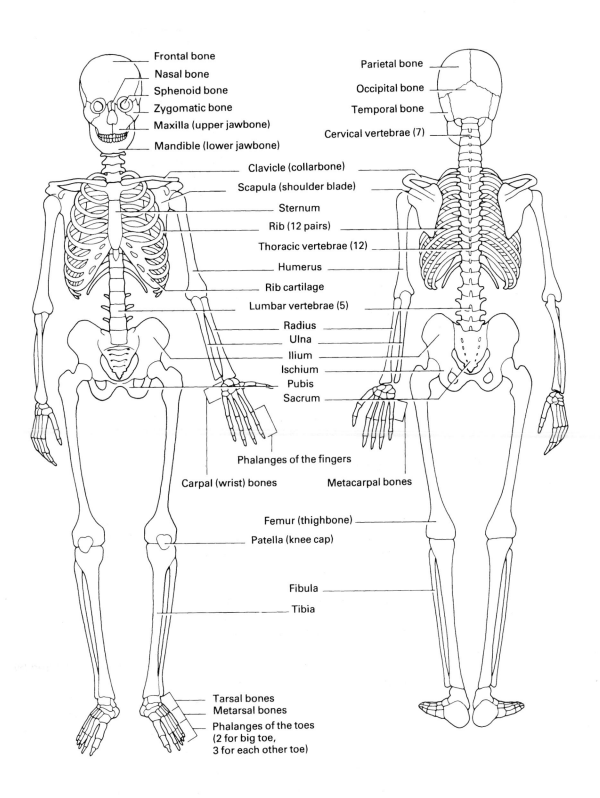

Frontal bone
Nasal bone
Sphenoid bone
Zygomatic bone
Maxilla (upper jawbone)
Mandible (lower jawbone)

Parietal bone
Occipital bone
Temporal bone
Cervical vertebrae (7)

Clavicle (collarbone)
Scapula (shoulder blade)
Sternum
Rib (12 pairs)
Thoracic vertebrae (12)
Humerus
Rib cartilage
Lumbar vertebrae (5)
Radius
Ulna
Ilium
Ischium
Pubis
Sacrum

Phalanges of the fingers

Carpal (wrist) bones   Metacarpal bones

Femur (thighbone)
Patella (knee cap)

Fibula
Tibia

Tarsal bones
Metatarsal bones
Phalanges of the toes
(2 for big toe,
3 for each other toe)

THE SKELETON

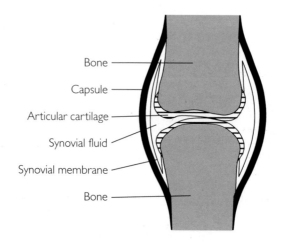

Bone

Capsule

Articular cartilage

Synovial fluid

Synovial membrane

Bone

A SECTION THROUGH A FREELY MOVABLE JOINT

The knee joint is the only articulation in the body which forms a full hinge, that is, the bones are capable of moving in either forward or backward directions. In practice this is prevented by the patella or kneecap which fits into the hinge rather like a doorstop or wedge. When the patella is not present, for example when it has been broken in an accident, the lower leg comes forward.

The capsule of the freely movable joints possesses small sacs containing a clear, viscous fluid. These structures which are called *mucous bursae* secrete synovial fluid. If the synovial membrane becomes inflamed this is known as *synovitis*. If the bursae become inflamed this is known as *bursitis*; the best known example of this is housemaid's knee – an occupational hazard for people whose work involves a good deal of kneeling.

Distribution of bones in the skeleton

The skull   The skull is made up of 22 bones, of which eight form the *cranium*:

- 1 frontal bone forming the forehead
- 2 parietal bones forming the top and sides of the cranium
- 1 occipital bone
- 2 temporal bones
- 1 sphenoid bone
- 1 ethmoid bone

and 14 form the *face* – the principal bones of which are:

- the superior maxilla or upper jaw
- the mandible or lower jaw (the jawbone which moves)
- 2 zygomatic or cheek bones
- 2 nasal bones which form the bridge of the nose
- 2 lacrimal bones.

16

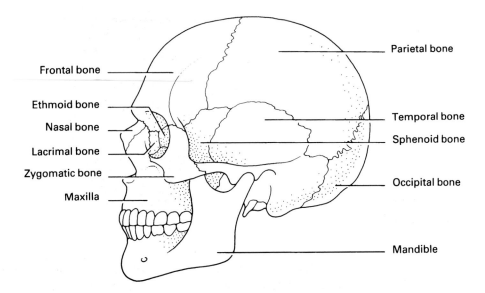

Frontal bone

Ethmoid bone

Nasal bone

Lacrimal bone

Zygomatic bone

Maxilla

Parietal bone

Temporal bone

Sphenoid bone

Occipital bone

Mandible

THE SKULL (SIDE VIEW)

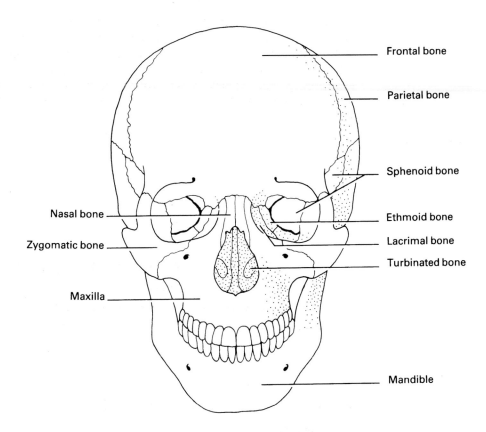

Frontal bone

Parietal bone

Nasal bone

Zygomatic bone

Maxilla

Sphenoid bone

Ethmoid bone

Lacrimal bone

Turbinated bone

Mandible

THE SKULL (ANTERIOR VIEW)

17

The thorax   Twenty-five bones form the thorax (or chest):

- the sternum or breast bone
- 12 pairs of ribs.

The first seven pairs are known as *true ribs* because each rib is joined to the sternum directly. The next five pairs (8th–12th) are known as *false ribs* because they do not join the sternum directly. The 8th, 9th and 10th ribs fuse with the rib immediately above, while the 11th and 12th pairs (*floating ribs*) only partly surround the circumference of the thorax and are unattached in front.

The spine   Thirty-three bones form the spine:

- 24 *true* or *movable* vertebrae, separated by pads of fibrocartilage
- 9 *false* or *fixed* vertebrae, closely fused together with no movement between them except the coccyx which moves with respect to the sacrum.

From the top of the spine downwards there are:

- 7 cervical vertebrae – the first is the atlas bone, the second is the axis bone
- 12 thoracic vertebrae
- 5 lumbar vertebrae
- 5 sacral vertebrae – fused to form the sacrum
- 4 coccygeal vertebrae – fused to form the coccyx.

The shoulder girdle

Four bones form the shoulder girdle:
- 2 clavicles or collar bones
- 2 scapulae or shoulder blades.

The upper limbs

Sixty bones form the upper limbs, 30 bones in each whole arm:

- 1 humerus or upper arm
- 1 radius – the outer bone of the forearm
- 1 ulna – the inner bone of the forearm
- 8 carpal bones forming the wrist
- 5 metacarpal bones forming the hand, and
- 14 phalanges or finger bones.

The pelvis

The pelvis is formed by four bones:

- the right and left innominate bones (hip bones)
- the sacrum and coccyx already referred to as part of the spinal vertebrae.

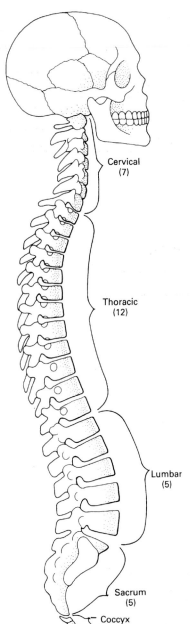

Cervical (7)

Thoracic (12)

Lumbar (5)

Sacrum (5)

Coccyx (4)

THE BONES OF THE SPINE

18

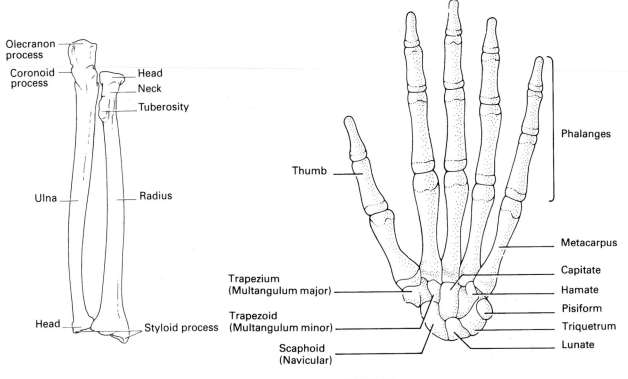

Olecranon process

Coronoid process

Head

Neck

Tuberosity

Ulna

Radius

Head

Styloid process

THE BONES OF THE FOREARM

Thumb

Phalanges

Metacarpus

Capitate

Hamate

Pisiform

Triquetrum

Lunate

Trapezium (Multangulum major)

Trapezoid (Multangulum minor)

Scaphoid (Navicular)

THE BONES OF THE LEFT HAND (ANTERIOR VIEW)

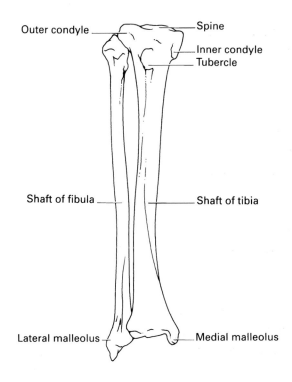

Outer condyle

Spine

Inner condyle

Tubercle

Shaft of fibula

Shaft of tibia

Lateral malleolus

Medial malleolus

BONES OF THE LOWER LEG

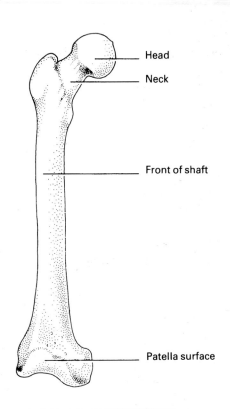

Head

Neck

Front of shaft

Patella surface

RIGHT FEMUR (ANTERIOR VIEW)

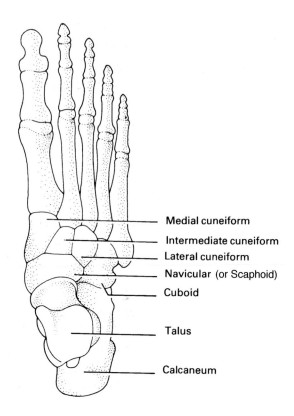

Medial cuneiform
Intermediate cuneiform
Lateral cuneiform
Navicular (or Scaphoid)
Cuboid

Talus

Calcaneum

THE BONES OF THE FOOT

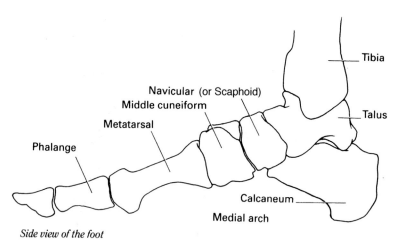

Navicular (or Scaphoid)
Middle cuneiform
Metatarsal
Phalange

Tibia

Talus

Calcaneum
Medial arch

THE BONES OF THE FOOT

Side view of the foot

Each innominate bone consists of:

- the ilium – upper portion
- the ischium – rear portion
- the pubis – front portion.

The lower limbs Sixty bones go to form the lower limbs, 30 in each whole leg:

- the femur or thigh bone
- the patella or kneecap

- the tibia or shin bone
- the fibula or brooch bone
- 7 tarsal bones of the ankle
- 5 metatarsal bones of the foot
- 14 phalanges of the toes.

In addition to the bones enumerated there is one hyoid bone which lies in the front upper part of the neck and is detached from the skeleton.

Spinal curvature

The illustration of the spine on page 18 shows that it has two natural curves – the slightly outward curving upper part of the spine being in the thoracic region, and the inward curving of the spine being in the lumbar region. These natural curvatures can be exaggerated by three basic causes:

- *congenital causes*, which are present at the time of birth or arising as a direct result of hereditary factors
- *traumatic causes*, resulting from accidents
- *environmental causes*, resulting from bad posture and often closely allied to the type of work in which a person is engaged.

There are three types of curvature of the spine:

- *kyphosis*, an exaggerated outward curvature of the spine
- *lordosis*, an inward exaggeration of the spine

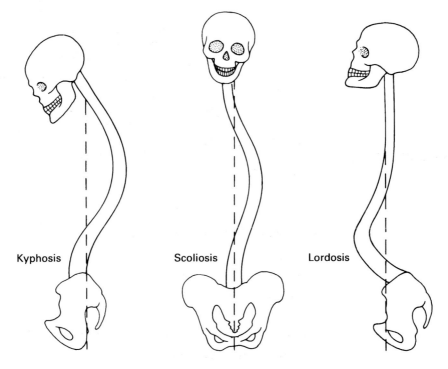

Kyphosis   Scoliosis   Lordosis

THE THREE TYPES OF CURVATURE OF THE SPINE

- *scoliosis*, a lateral curvature of the spine, which may occur at any part of the spine and is quite often associated with one of the other curvatures, e.g. the 'Hunchback of Notre Dame' suffered from kyphosis and scoliosis of the thoracic region.

Fractures

When a bone breaks it is referred to as a fracture. Fractures are divided into a number of categories:

- *simple fracture* when a bone breaks in one place and no serious damage is done to the surrounding tissues

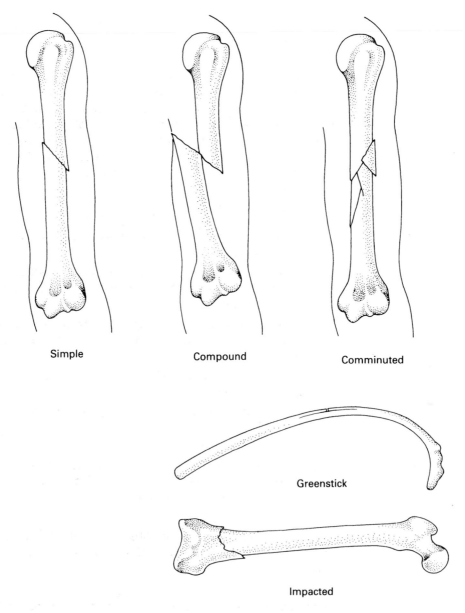

Simple   Compound   Comminuted

Greenstick

Impacted

THE TYPES OF FRACTURE

- *complicated fracture* when the bone is broken and the break causes injury of the surrounding soft tissue
- *compound fracture* when the bone is broken and one or both ends protrude through the external surface of the body, that is, through the skin
- *comminuted fracture* where the bone is broken in a number of places
- *impacted fracture* where the bone is broken and one end is driven into the other
- *greenstick fracture*, an incomplete fracture of a long bone as seen in young children.

Conditions and diseases of the skeletal system

Arthritis The skeleton is subject to many diseases, most of which do not come within the scope of this textbook. However, mention must be made of arthritis because it is such a universal disease. Technically arthritis is an inflammation of a joint but this is generally interpreted as being a rheumatic affection of the joint, i.e. the inflammation is caused by the type of rheumatism which primarily affects the skeletal system, as distinct from fibrositis and neuritis which are dealt with in later chapters.

There are many types of arthritis – among the more common being:

- *mono-articular arthritis*, which as the name implies, is a type of arthritis which involves only one joint
- *poly-articular arthritis*, which attacks a number of joints, usually associated joints, i.e. both hips or both knees or, in some cases, all the joints of one leg or arm
- *osteo- or degenerative arthritis*, which is a chronic joint disease characterised by loss of some of the joint's cartilage and some spur formation
- *rheumatoid arthritis*, which is a chronic arthritis usually associated with hormone deficiency
- *gouty arthritis* (see Glossary), which is popularly associated with the big toe.

Paget's disease Paget's disease (osteo deformens) is a relatively common bone disease in people over 40. It is a chronic process of bone overgrowth, destruction, and new bone formation.

Frozen shoulder Frozen shoulder (adhesive capsulitis) is not fully understood, but common causes include septic arthritis, rheumatoid arthritis and local trauma.

Tennis elbow Tennis elbow is an acute or chronic synovitis of the radiohumeral articulation.

23

The skeleton in rhyme

Learning and understanding the anatomical details of the skeleton is no easy task. The poem below, written by Amanda Cornford, may help you.

The human skeleton, you know, has very many bits
  When all the bones are added up they number two-0-six.
The axial make up 80, sternum, spine and skull and ribs –
  The rest are appendicular, shoulders, arms and legs and hips.

The skull itself has 22, each fixed in its own place.
  8 cranial bones protect the brain, and 14 form the face.
2 parietal bones on top, a frontal at the fore.
  2 temporal on either side connect up to the jaw.
The occipital bone behind makes contact with the spine
  The way each part connects is just a marvel of design.
The sphenoid is the keystone of the cranial template,
  and with the nasal ethmoid bone, these cranial bones make
    eight.

Now 14 bones make up the face, and some are very small.
  The lachrymal and nasal bones hardly show at all.
The vomer and 2 palatines, as G. Tortora shows,
  Contribute to the orbits, the hard palate and the nose.
2 maxillae unite to form a single upper jaw
  With the zygomatic cheekbones, that makes another four.
The mandible or lower jaw's the largest, strongest bone
  It's the only facial one to move – in this, it stands alone.

The skull sits on a column of stacked up vertebrae.
  The number of these knobbly bones amounts to 33.
There are 7 cervical bones that constitute the neck,
  And 12 thoracic vertebrae attached to ribs, just check!
The 5 lumbar vertebrae are the strongest of them all.
  The sacrum is 5 vertebrae, fused to make one wall.
The coccyx too is 4 fused bones, the tail end of the spine
  And all these bones, all 33, make one long curving line.
12 pairs of ribs, 7 true, 5 false, are fastened to this column
  And all but 4 attach in front to the breastbone called the
    sternum.
All 25 of these chest bones play an important part
  They form the thoracic cavity which houses lungs and
    heart.

The remainder of the body's bones are appendicular
  Of which the thigh, or femur, is the strongest one by far.
I'll tell you now quite briefly how the pectoral girdle's made,
  How the clavicle, or collar bone, joins to the shoulder blade.
They meet at the acromion, the flat end of the spine
  Which runs across the shoulder blade in an unbroken line.

This shoulder blade, or scapula's triangular and flat.
    It's held in its position by the muscles of the back.
Beneath the joint acromial a shallow hollow lurks;
    Here in this glenoid cavity the humerus inserts.
The clavicle, as you may know, on the anterior side,
    Attaches to the sternum, at the manubrium divide.

2 scapulae, 2 clavicles, these bones thus number four.
    With 30 bones per arm and hand that makes for 60 more.
The humerus or arm bone from the shoulder joint depends
    The radius and the ulna bones the upper arm extend.
The ulna is the medial bone, the longest of the pair.
    Its head is known as funny bone, or elbow, I declare.
Beneath this knobbly process, olecranon as it's called,
    Is a notch in which the trochlea of the upper arm's installed.
The radius is the lateral bone which to the wrist connects
    By the lunate and the scaphoid bones, just where the thumb
       projects.
These two small bones are carpal bones, of which the total's eight.
    Trapezium, triquetrum, trapezoid and capitate,
With hamate bone and pisiform make up the final score.
    The carpals with the tarsals when compared have one bone more.
5 metacarpals form the palm, and phalanges 14,
    Or finger bones, as they are known, complete our brachial scene.

2 nameless bones, innominates, the pelvic girdle form,
    For each an ilium, ischium and pelvis is the norm.
The jutting hip bone you can feel is called the ileac crest,
    The sacroiliac joint nearby can sometimes cause distress. The
ischial tuberosities are what you sit upon
    The pelvis joins the other parts at the acetabulum.
This socket holds the femur, or strong bone of the thigh,
    Which hinges with the tibia, or shin bone, bye the bye.
This hinge is called the knee joint and it has a small round cap
    A sesamoid bone called patella, which doctors like to tap.
The tibia is supported, along its lateral length,
    By the fibula, or brooch bone, which lends additional strength.
Both tibia and fibula make contact with the talus,
    And this in turn impinges on the heel, calcaneus.
The bones that go to make the foot amount to 6 and 20,
    7 tarsal bones, 5 metatarsals and phalanges aplenty.

3 auditory ossicles exist in either ear,
    But if you start to count those in you'll get confused I fear.
But don't forget the Y shaped bone, which I must not avoid
    Informing you about, and that's the throat bone, or hyoid.
By certain counts this bone is not included in
    The 206 we started with, but that is not a sin.
These lines should help remind you when the ITEC test is here
    Provided you don't panic then, you should have nought to fear!

GLOSSARY

Acromion	a flat, rather triangular bony process formed by the lateral extension of the scapula spine
Appendicular skeleton	skeleton of the upper and lower limbs and their girdles
Axial skeleton	skeleton of the head and trunk
Cancellous tissue	characterised by a latticed structure as seen in the spongy tissue of bones
Cartilage	a substance similar to bone but not as hard. It acts as a cushion between bones and also gives shape to nose and ears.
Condyle	a rounded eminence of bones forming joints, e.g. femur, humerus
Dislocation	occurs when force is applied to a joint and is greater than that necessary to produce a strain. It particularly applies to ball and socket joints as the ball is forced out of the socket. When dislocated bones are returned to their proper position this is referred to as *reduction*.
Glenoid cavity	a shallow cavity usually associated with the shoulder joint
Gouty arthritis	occurs in any part of the body but is popularly associated with the big toe. It results from urate crystals (chalky salts of uric acid) being deposited in and around the cartilage. This form of arthritis is much more common in men than women.
Hyoid	sometimes called the hyoid bone, but more accurately ossified cartilage, between the root of the tongue and the larynx
Manubrium	the first or upper part of the sternum
Oleocranon	the point of the elbow
Orthopaedics	branch of surgery concerned with corrective treatment of skeletal system
Ossicle	a small bone, e.g. the malleus
Osteo	referring to bone
Periosteum	the hard membrane adhering to a bone and forming a protective cover. It contains blood vessels supplying blood to the bone and at its deepest layers are the bone-forming cells – osteoblasts.
Rickets	a calcium deficiency disease of children usually evidenced by misshapen bones
Spondylitis	a type of arthritis which attacks the spinal vertebrae; the severest form is *ankylosing spondylitis* where bone and cartilage fuse resulting in complete immobility
Tuberosity	a protuberance on a bone

4 The Muscular System

The main framework of the skeleton of the body is covered by muscles. These are responsible for 50 per cent of our body weight and their function is to permit movement, for which purpose they are, in most cases, attached to bones.

There are two types of muscle:

- *voluntary muscles*, which are under conscious control, such as those used in walking or writing
- *involuntary muscles*, which are outside conscious control, such as those which are involved in the movement of the heart, respiration and digestion.

A section of voluntary muscle shows it to be of striped and striated (cross-banded) tissue, whilst involuntary muscles have slender, smooth types of cells without cross stripes and are therefore usually referred to as smooth muscles.

A section of *cardiac* (heart) muscle tissue shows that, whilst it is involuntary muscle, it has characteristics which bear a superficial resemblance to voluntary muscle tissue though the fibres are smaller than those of voluntary muscles and the striae are not so well marked.

A muscle consists of a number of contractile or elastic fibres bound together in bundles. The bundles are, in turn, bound together by a thick band usually spindle-shaped and always contained in a sheath. This sheath is extended at the end to form strong fibrous bands known as the tendons by means of which the muscles are fastened to the bones.

Altogether there are some 640 named muscles in the body but there are many, many thousands of unnamed ones – each hair on the surface of the body having a tiny muscle attached to it. When a person gets chilled or frightened and has what are known as 'goose pimples' – the little lumps on the skin are due to the tiny muscles of the skin pulling the hair erect. Muscles are well supplied with arteries to bring them food for fuel and repair, and oxygen for combustion of the fuel, and with veins which carry away the waste products of their activities, such as carbon dioxide.

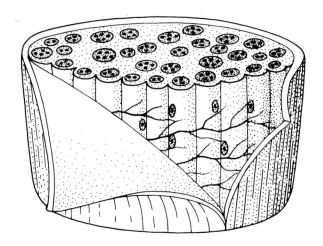

A CROSS-SECTION THROUGH
A MUSCLE

How muscles work

The muscles which are responsible for skeletal movements have two points of attachment – the *point of origin* is the bone to which they are attached and which they *do not* move and the *point of insertion* is the bone to which they are attached and which they *do* move, e.g. the biceps of the arm has its point of origin at the shoulder end of the arm, whilst the point of insertion is the radius of the lower arm. Therefore it is the lower arm that is activated by the biceps.

A muscle receives its stimulus from a motor nerve and in response to this stimulus it shortens its length so that, *in action*, a muscle always contracts. Muscles in the body normally work in pairs. One is the *prime mover* and the other one holds it in check. This means that the voluntary muscles are never completely at rest. They are normally in a condition of slight tension or contraction and this we call *muscular tone*.

When one or more muscles are active in the initiation and maintenance of a movement they are called *prime movers* and when one or more muscles wholly oppose this they are referred to as *antagonists*. For example, when we bend our forearm, the muscles on the front of the arm contract whilst, at the same time, the muscles on the back of the arm relax gradually to maintain balance. In this instance the muscles at the front of the arm are the prime movers, whilst the ones at the back are the antagonists. However, to reverse this position and straighten the arm out again the muscles on the back of the arm become the prime movers and those on the front become the antagonists.

Muscles are put into groups according to the functions which they perform:

- An *extensor* extends a limb.
- A *flexor* flexes a limb.
- An *adductor* bends a limb towards the median line.
- An *abductor* takes a limb away from the median line.
- A *sphincter* surrounds and closes an orifice or opening.

28

- A *supinator* turns a limb to face upwards.
- A *pronator* turns a limb to face downwards.
- *Rotators* rotate a limb.

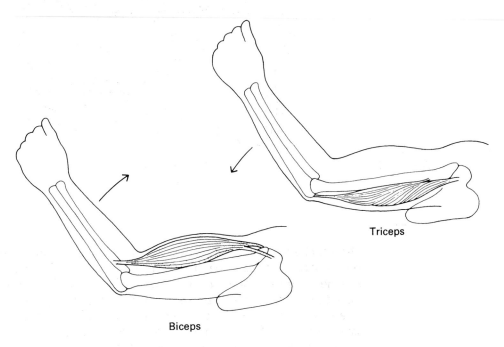

Triceps

Biceps

AN EXAMPLE OF A FLEXOR MUSCLE   AN EXAMPLE OF AN EXTENSOR MUSCLE

Muscular activity also contributes materially to the internal heat of the body and when there is a danger of this reaching too low a level a person shivers. This is an involuntary action making the muscles work in order to generate more heat. Muscles are, in turn, responsive to exterior heat so that exposure of the skin to cold air increases muscle tone whereas considerable heat, e.g. a hot bath, has a relaxing effect on muscles. About 30 per cent of the energy produced in muscle activity results in work and the remaining 70 per cent is released as heat which warms the body, particularly the blood.

As previously mentioned, muscle contraction occurs as the result of a stimulus which it receives from a motor nerve. This nerve stimulus sets up chemical changes in the muscles. These changes include the breaking down of glucose, glycogen and fat, which, in turn, liberate the energy required for contraction. In the process of contraction there are some waste products which are excreted from the muscles by the venous system. However, if at any one time the muscular activity is so great as to produce more waste products than the venous and lymph systems are able to cope with, then some waste products remain in the muscle or between the muscle fibres and give a feeling of stiffness – that is the fibres are no longer easily able to slide one over the other.

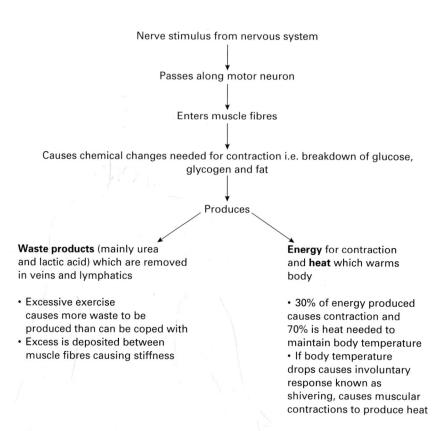

Nerve stimulus from nervous system

Passes along motor neuron

Enters muscle fibres

Causes chemical changes needed for contraction i.e. breakdown of glucose, glycogen and fat

Produces

Waste products (mainly urea and lactic acid) which are removed in veins and lymphatics

• Excessive exercise causes more waste to be produced than can be coped with
• Excess is deposited between muscle fibres causing stiffness

Energy for contraction and **heat** which warms body

• 30% of energy produced causes contraction and 70% is heat needed to maintain body temperature
• If body temperature drops causes involuntary response known as shivering, causes muscular contractions to produce heat

MUSCULAR CONTRACTION

Principal muscles in the body

The following tables (pages 33, 34, 36 and 37) list some of the principal muscles of the body. This is by no means a complete list and students who wish to study the subject in greater depth as well as to learn the origins and insertions of muscles are referred to one of the standard anatomical textbooks dealing with this subject. But this list should cover most, if not all, of the muscles that the physical therapist is likely to have to deal with.

Muscles printed in bold type are illustrated in the diagrams.

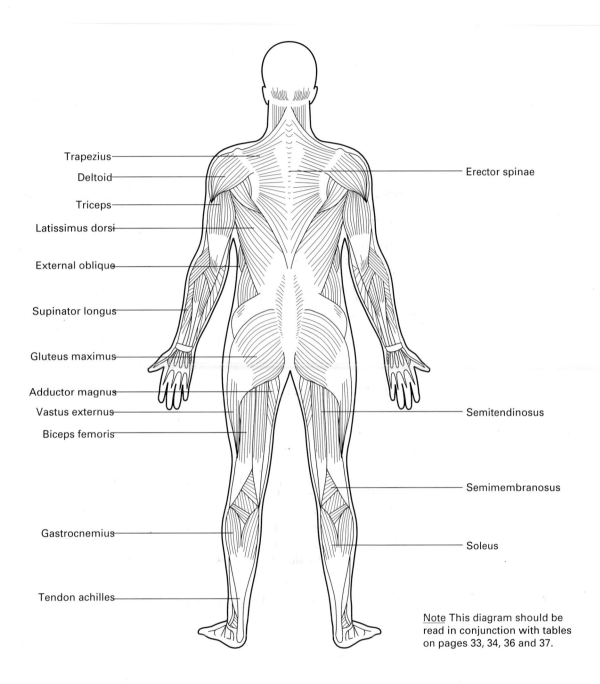

Trapezius

Deltoid

Triceps

Latissimus dorsi

External oblique

Supinator longus

Gluteus maximus

Adductor magnus

Vastus externus

Biceps femoris

Gastrocnemius

Tendon achilles

Erector spinae

Semitendinosus

Semimembranosus

Soleus

Note This diagram should be read in conjunction with tables on pages 33, 34, 36 and 37.

MUSCLES OF THE BODY (POSTERIOR VIEW)

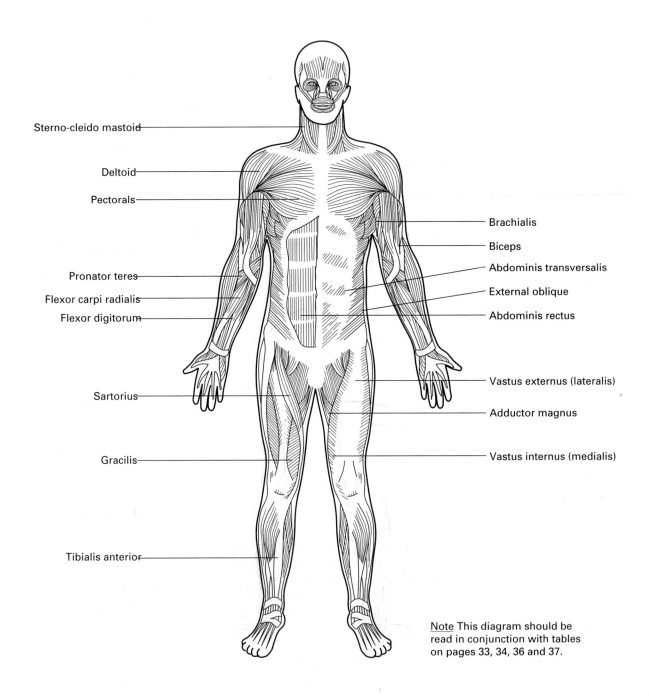

Sterno-cleido mastoid

Deltoid

Pectorals

Brachialis

Biceps

Abdominis transversalis

Pronator teres

External oblique

Flexor carpi radialis

Abdominis rectus

Flexor digitorum

Vastus externus (lateralis)

Sartorius

Adductor magnus

Gracilis

Vastus internus (medialis)

Tibialis anterior

<u>Note</u> This diagram should be read in conjunction with tables on pages 33, 34, 36 and 37.

MUSCLES OF THE BODY (ANTERIOR VIEW)

Muscles of the head and neck

Name	Action	Point of origin	Point of insertion
Epicraneas	Elevates eyebrows and draws scalp forward	Occipital and frontal bones	Aponeurosis of scalp
Orbicularis oculi	Closes eyelids	Frontal bone	Frontal process of maxilla
Oribicularis oris	Puckers mouth	No bone attachments	
Masseter	Muscle of mastication, closes mouth, clenches teeth	Zygomatic arch	Mandible
Buccinator	Compresses cheeks and retracts angle of mouth	Maxilla and mandible	Corner of mouth
Sterno-cleido mastoid (Sterno-mastoid)	Flexes head and turns from side to side	Sternum and clavicle	Mastoid process of temporal bone
Platysma	Muscle of facial expression	Fascia of pectoralis and deltoid	Mandible

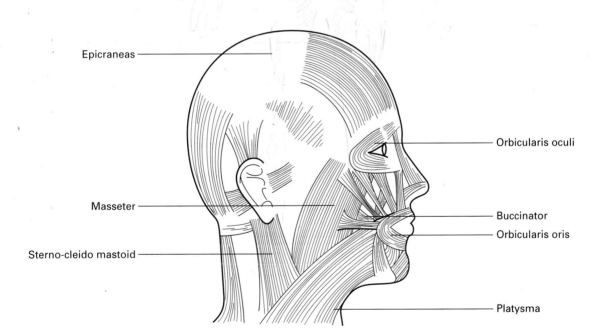

THE MUSCLES OF THE HEAD AND NECK

Muscles of the trunk of the body

Name	Action	Point of Origin	Point of insertion
Trapezius	Rotates inferior angle of scapula laterally, raises shoulder, draws scapula backwards	Occipital and spines of thoracic vertebra	Clavicle and spine of scapula
Erector spinae	Extends vertebral column	Sacrum	Occipital bone
Splenius capitis	Extends head	Spines of last cervical and upper thoracic vertebrae	Mastoid process
Latissimus dorsi	Adducts the shoulder and extends humerus. Used to pull body up in climbing	Lumbar vertebra, sacrum and iliac crest	Humerus
Serratus anterior (Serratus magnus)	Draws the scapula forward	Upper nine ribs	Vertebral border of scapula
Gluteus maximus	Extends hip joint and extends trunk on buttocks in raising body from sitting position	Ilium, sacrum and coccyx	Upper end of femur
Psoas	Flexes hip joint and trunk on lower extremities	Lumbar vertebra	Femur
Pectoralis major	Flexes shoulder joint, depresses shoulder girdle, adducts and rotates humerus	Sternum and clavicle	Humerus
Abdominis obliquus (internal and external oblique)	Supports abdominal viscera and flexes vertebral column	Lower ribs and iliac crest	Iliac crest and lower ribs
Abdominis transversalis (transversus abdominis)	Supports abdominal viscera and flexes vertebral column	Costal cartilages of 6 ribs and iliac crest	Linea alba and pubic bone
Abdominis rectus	Supports abdominal viscera and flexes vertebral column	Upper border of pubic bone	5th to 7th costal cartilage
Rhomboids	Draws scapula backwards	Vertebral scapula	Dorsal scapula
Infraspinalis	Rotates humerus	Scapula	Humerus
Supraspinalis	Abducts humerus	Scapula	Humerus
Teres major	Adducts humerus	Scapula	Humerus
Teres minor	Rotates humerus	Scapula	Humerus
Gluteus medius	Abducts femur	Ilium (pelvis)	Femur

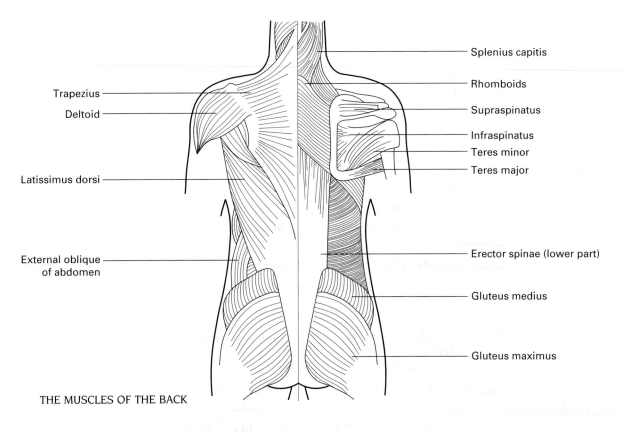

Trapezius

Deltoid

Latissimus dorsi

External oblique
of abdomen

Splenius capitis

Rhomboids

Supraspinatus

Infraspinatus

Teres minor

Teres major

Erector spinae (lower part)

Gluteus medius

Gluteus maximus

THE MUSCLES OF THE BACK

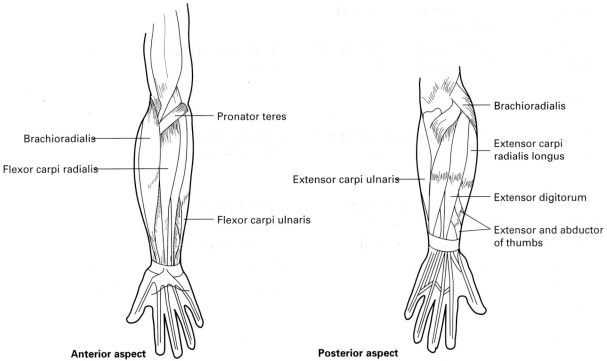

Brachioradialis

Flexor carpi radialis

Pronator teres

Flexor carpi ulnaris

Anterior aspect

Brachioradialis

Extensor carpi
radialis longus

Extensor carpi ulnaris

Extensor digitorum

Extensor and abductor
of thumbs

Posterior aspect

THE SUPERFICIAL MUSCLES OF THE FOREARM

Muscles of the arms

Name	Action	Point of origin	Point of insertion
Deltoid	Abduction of the humerus to right angle	Spine of scapula and clavicle	Humerus
Biceps brachialis	Flexes and supinates forearm	Scapula	Radial tuberosity
Triceps brachialis	Extends elbow joint	Scapula and humerus	Ulna
Brachialis	Flexes elbow joint	Humerus	Ulna
Coraco brachialis	Flexes and adducts humerus	Scapula	Humerus
Brachioradialis (supinator longus)	Flexes elbow joint	Humerus	Radius
Pronator teres (pronator radii teres)	Pronates forearm	Humerus and ulna	Radius
Supinator (supinator radii brevis)	Supinates forearm	Humerus	Radius
Flexor carpi radialis	Flexes wrist joint	Humerus	Second metacarpal
Extensor carpi (radialis longus)	Extends wrists	Humerus	Base of second metacarpal
Flexor carpi ulnaris	Flexes wrist joint	Humerus and border of ulna	Fifth metacarpal
Extensor carpi ulnaris	Extends wrist joint	Humerus and ulna	Base of fifth metacarpal
Flexor digitorum	Flexes fingers	Ulna	Four tendons to base of each finger
Extensor digitorum	Extends fingers	Humerus	Four extensor tendons of each finger

Muscles of the legs

Name	Action	Point of origin	Point of insertion
Rectus femoris (Quadriceps)	Extends knee joint	Ilium	Upper border patella
Vastus laterialis (externus) (Quadriceps)	Extends knee joint	Femur	Tibia
Vastus medialis (internus) (Quadriceps)	Extends knee joint	Femur	Tibia
Vastus intermedius (Quadriceps)	Extends knee joint	Femur	Tibia
Semitendinosus (hamstring)	Flexes knee joint and extends hip joint	Ischium (of pelvis)	Tibia
Semi-membranosus (hamstring)	Flexes knee joint and extends hip joint	Ischium (of pelvis)	Tibia
Gracilis	Adducts femur and flexes knee joint	Pubis	Tibia
Gastrocnemius	Flexes ankle and knee joint	Femur	Tendon of achilles and calcaneum
Tibialis anterior (tibialis anticus)	Extends and inverts foot	Tibia	Cuneiform and 1st metatarsal
Peroneus longus	Inverts and flexes foot and supports arches	Tibia and fibula	Cuneiform and 1st metatarsal
Flexor digitorum longus	Flexes toes	Tibia	Four tendons to base of each toe
Extensor digitorum longus	Extends toes	Tibia and fibula	Extensor tendon on each toe
Tendon of achilles	Assists in flexion of the foot	Gastrocnemius and soleus	Heel of foot
Soleus	Flexes ankle joint	Tibia and fibula	Calcaneum
Sartorius	Flexes hip and knee joint and rotates femur laterally	Iliac spine	Tibia
Biceps femoris (hamstring)	Flexes knee joint	Femur	Fibula
Adductor magnus, longus and brevis	Adducts thigh	Pubis	Femur

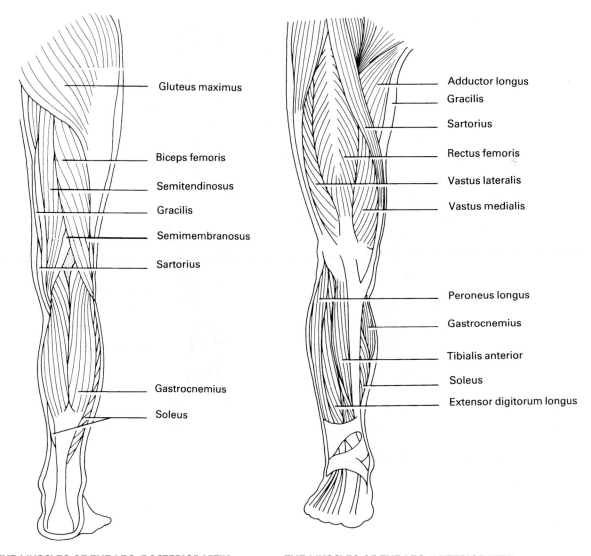

THE MUSCLES OF THE LEG (POSTERIOR VIEW)   THE MUSCLES OF THE LEG (ANTERIOR VIEW)

Common diseases or conditions of the muscular system

Fibrositis   This is one of the most common diseases of the muscular system. Fibrositis means inflammation of soft tissue and is a term which is generally applied to a rheumatic affection of the muscles – a condition in which there is a build-up of urea and lactic acid inside the muscle to the extent of causing stiffness and pain.

A well known example of this disease is *lumbago* or fibrositis of muscles in the lumbar region. *Torticollis* or 'wry neck' is another condition which has much in common with muscular fibrositis, in this case the muscle concerned in the sterno-cleido mastoid muscle of the neck which, in a state of contraction, causes the head to take up an abnormal position.

38

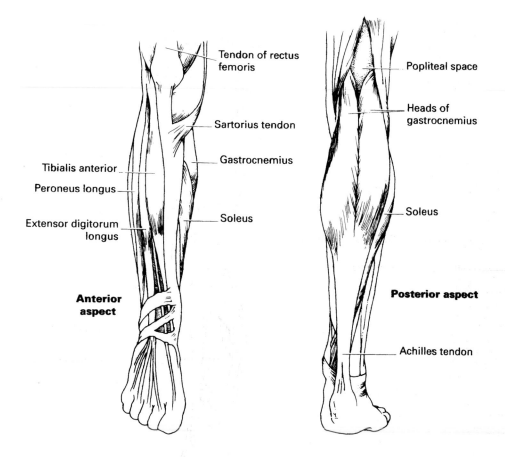

Tendon of rectus femoris

Popliteal space

Heads of gastrocnemius

Sartorius tendon

Gastrocnemius

Tibialis anterior

Peroneus longus

Soleus

Extensor digitorum longus

Soleus

Anterior aspect

Posterior aspect

Achilles tendon

THE SUPERFICIAL MUSCLES OF THE LOWER LEG

Cramp   This is a localised painful contraction of one or more muscles, which has a number of causes, the most usual being that of vigorous exercise; but it also occurs in certain metabolic disorders, e.g. when there is a sodium depletion or water depletion. It is for the purpose of avoiding cramp that copious quantities of salted water are given to people who work in intense heat – for example, people who look after furnaces at steelworks.

Muscle fatigue   This is usually caused by sustained or repeated muscular contractions. In this condition, the muscles suffer from a lack of glycogen and fluid and a build-up of lactic acid. This results in diminished capacity to respond to stimulation.

There are also conditions which affect muscles but whose cause is to be found in one of the other systems. For example, *poliomyelitis* (commonly called 'polio') which arises in the neurological system, and *multiple* or *disseminated sclerosis* which also arises in the neurological system. Both these conditions profoundly affect the body's musculature.

GLOSSARY

Atony	abnormally low degree of tonus or absence of it
Atrophy	reduction in the size of a muscle which previously reached a matured size; popularly referred to as wastage
Cramp	painful involuntary contraction of muscle
Fascia	the sheath or membrane covering a muscle
Ganglion	a cystic swelling which occurs in association with a joint or tendon sheath. Ganglia most commonly occur on the back of the wrist
Myology	the science of muscles
Myositis	inflammation of a muscle
Ligaments	bands of fibrous tissue which help to bind the bones of joints together
Rupture	a tearing or bursting of the fascia or sheath which surrounds the fibres of the muscles
Spasm	a sudden muscular contraction
Spastic	pertaining to or characterised by spasm; once commonly used in reference to cerebral palsy
Sprain	an injury to a ligament
Strain	an injury to a muscle or its tendon
Tendon	a band of fibrous tissue forming the end of a muscle and attaching it to the bone
Tonus	muscle tone
Viscera	the contents of the abdominal cavity

5 The Vascular System

The vascular system, which is sometimes called the circulatory system, consists of the heart, blood vessels, blood, lymphatic vessels and lymph.

The heart

The centre of the vascular system is the *heart*, which is a muscular organ that rhythmically contracts, forcing the blood through a system of vessels. The heart weighs approximately 255 g in a fully grown adult and lies one-third to the right and two-thirds to the left of the thoracic cavity. At birth it beats about 130 times a minute, at six years about 100 times a minute, reducing in adult life to between 65 and 80 beats a minute with an average somewhere around 70. During a 24-hour period an adult human heart pumps 36 000 litres of blood through the 20 000 km of blood vessels.

The heart is divided into four chambers. These are the *right and the left atria* (or *auricles*), in the upper part of the heart, and the *right and left ventricles* in the lower part. The right side of the heart is divided from the

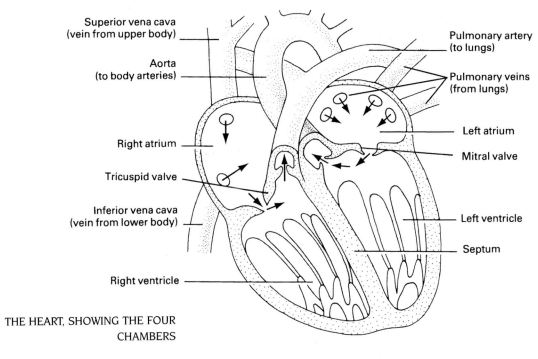

Superior vena cava (vein from upper body)

Aorta (to body arteries)

Right atrium

Tricuspid valve

Inferior vena cava (vein from lower body)

Right ventricle

Pulmonary artery (to lungs)

Pulmonary veins (from lungs)

Left atrium

Mitral valve

Left ventricle

Septum

THE HEART, SHOWING THE FOUR CHAMBERS

left by a solid wall called the *septum* which prevents the venous blood on the right side coming into contact with the arterial blood on the left side of the heart.

Circulation is divided into two principal systems: the *general* or *systemic circulation* (around the body); and the *pulmonary circulation* (to and from the lungs).

The general circulation includes two special branches: the *portal circulation*, which conveys blood from the digestive organs to the liver; and the *coronary circulation*, which supplies the heart.

Arteries and veins

Blood vessels which proceed from the heart are known as *arteries*. They generally carry oxygenated blood (the exception being the pulmonary artery). They are large, hollow, elastic tubes which gradually decrease in diameter as they spread through the body. These smaller arteries finally become very fine hairlike vessels known as *capillaries*.

Blood vessels which proceed towards the heart are known as *veins*. They generally carry deoxygenated blood (the exception being the pulmonary vein). They are elastic tubes with valves which prevent a backward flow of blood.

The veins empty the deoxygenated blood into the right atrium of the heart from the *inferior* and *superior vena cava*. The blood flows through the *tricuspid valve* to the right ventricle and is pumped to the lungs via the pulmonary artery. This is the only artery in the body to carry deoxygenated blood.

The blood is reoxygenated in the lungs and returns to the left atrium of the heart through the pulmonary veins. These are the only veins to transport oxygenated blood. The blood flows into the left ventricle through the *mitral valve* and is pumped to the body through the *aorta*.

The aorta is the largest artery in the body. It has two branches: the ascending aorta, supplying the arms and head; and the descending aorta, supplying the lower part of the body.

The descending aorta passes from the thorax through the diaphragm to the abdomen, where it is called the *abdominal aorta*. The *coeliac axis*, which branches off the abdominal aorta, supplies the stomach, liver and spleen. Below this the *renal arteries* branch off to the kidneys and the *mesenteric arteries* to the intestines. Finally the abdominal aorta branches into two *iliac arteries* which run into the pelvis. The *internal iliac artery* supplies the reproductive organs while the *external iliac artery* becomes the *femoral artery* which is the main artery of the lower limb.

The femoral artery supplies the thigh muscles and becomes the *popliteal artery* at the knee. This divides into the *anterior* and *posterior tibial arteries*. The anterior tibial artery supplies the front of the leg and is continued to the foot as the *dorsalis pedis artery*. The posterior tibial artery supplies the back of the leg and reaches the sole of the foot as the *plantar artery* which forms the *plantar arches*.

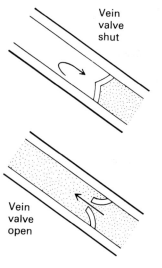

Vein valve shut

Vein valve open

VEINS (CONVEY BLOOD TO THE HEART)

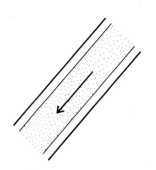

ARTERY (CONVEYS BLOOD AWAY FROM THE HEART)

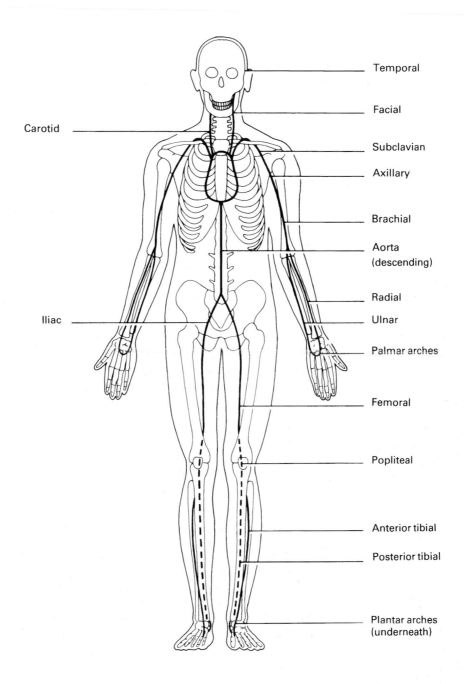

Temporal

Facial

Carotid

Subclavian

Axillary

Brachial

Aorta
(descending)

Radial

Ulnar

Iliac

Palmar arches

Femoral

Popliteal

Anterior tibial

Posterior tibial

Plantar arches
(underneath)

THE ARTERIES OF THE BODY

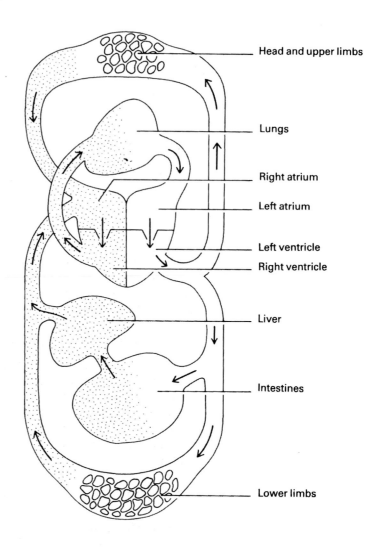

Head and upper limbs

Lungs

Right atrium

Left atrium

Left ventricle

Right ventricle

Liver

Intestines

Lower limbs

THE DIRECTION OF CIRCULATION

Two *coronary arteries* branch off the ascending aorta, which then passes upwards as the *innominate artery*. This divides into the *subclavian* and *carotid arteries*.

The subclavian artery passes behind the clavicle and enters the armpit where it becomes the *axillary artery*. The *brachial artery* continues for the length of the upper arm until the elbow where it divides into the *radial* and *ulnar arteries*, culminating in the *palmar arches* in the hand.

The carotid artery passes upwards to the neck and has four main branches, the *facial, temporal, occipital* and *maxillary arteries*.

Blood

The composition of blood

Blood is alkaline in reaction and amounts to approximately 4–5 litres in the average adult. It is complex in nature but has four principal constituent parts:

- *plasma*
- *erythrocytes* (red corpuscles)
- *leucocytes* (white corpuscles)
- *platelets*.

Plasma

Plasma provides the liquid basis of the blood. It is a clear, straw-coloured liquid which holds various substances in solution. These include sugar, urea, amino acids, mineral salts, enzymes, etc.

Erythrocytes

Erythrocytes or red corpuscles (corpuscles is Latin for little bodies) are inert biconcave discs. They get their colour from haemoglobin which has the ability to absorb oxygen (when it becomes *oxy-haemoglobin* which is bright red in colour) and carbon dioxide (when it becomes *carboxy-haemoglobin* which becomes very dark red, bordering on a muddy brown colour). The average life span of an erythrocyte is 120 days. They are produced mainly in red bone marrow and their eventual disintegration takes place in the spleen, and is finally completed in the liver.

In health, the erythrocytes total about 5 million per cubic millimetre of blood which gives a total of somewhere in the region of 25 billion in a human adult. If these cells were placed end to end they would form a ribbon sufficiently long to encircle the world more than four times. These cells are the body's transporters; they carry oxygen to all parts of the body and on their return journey pick up waste products, primarily carbon dioxide.

Leucocytes

Leucocytes or phagocytes (white corpuscles) are larger than erythrocytes and have an irregular shape and a nucleus. They are produced in the bone marrow and, in health, they total about 8000 per cubic millimetre. They are the protectors or soldiers of the body; their chief role is to protect the body against infection by their power of ingesting bacteria – a process which is known as *phagocytosis*. When the body is subject to serious infection the leucocytes increase rapidly by a process of division known as *mitosis*.

Platelets

Platelets or *thrombocytes* average 250 000 per cubic millimetre of blood. They are derived from large multi-nucleated cells in the bone marrow and are essential to the blood for coagulation, i.e. clotting.

Put simply, when a cut or abrasion exposes blood to the air, the combination of thrombocytes, fibrinogen and air forms a clot. However, the clotting process can be much more complicated, especially when the clotting takes place within the body, e.g. thrombophlebitis. This happens when the fibrinogen level exceeds the norm. The thrombocytes, having produced excess thrombokinase, act on prothrombin (already in the blood) to change it to thrombin which, after reaction with calcium ions, results in the over-production of fibrinogen.

The spleen

The spleen lies below the left dome of the diaphragm, literally on top of the liver, but smaller than it. It is covered entirely by the ribs within a fibrous capsule. It is soft, vascular and is bluish-red in colour.

The function of the spleen is to serve as a reservoir of erythrocytes, and in addition it produces antibodies and lymphocytes. A further function is to remove from the circulatory system worn-out erythrocytes, thrombocytes and leucocytes. Sometimes, as a result of accidents, it is necessary to remove the spleen when it appears that other parts of the body are able to take over its functions.

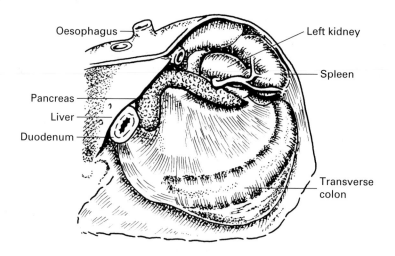

THE POSITION OF THE SPLEEN

Blood types The existence of human blood types was established by Karl Landsteiner in 1902 when he began a study to determine why fatalities occurred following some blood transfusions. He discovered that the cause was incompatibility between the blood of the donor and the blood of the recipient.

Arising from this work came the Landsteiner Classification of Blood Groups which classified blood into the four types A, B, AB and O.

Type O is called the *universal donor* because it may give blood to all blood types, but it can only receive from type O. On the other hand, type AB is called the *universal recipient* because it can receive from any group, but can only give to the AB group. Type A can give to both A and AB and receive only from types A and O. Type B can give to types B and AB and receive only from types B or O.

In 1940 Landsteiner and A. S. Weiner recognised the Rh factor, a substance found in red blood cells. This was discovered during their experiments with rhesus monkeys, hence the name rhesus or the abbreviation Rh. It is estimated that 85 per cent of white people have Rh positive factor and the other 15 per cent are Rh negative.

Blood pressure The blood in the circulatory system is always under pressure, which depends on:

- the amount of blood in the system
- the strength and rate of the heart's contractions
- the elasticity of the arteries.

Doctors measure two phases of blood pressure:

- *systolic pressure*, which is the blood pressure when the heart is contracted
- *diastolic pressure*, which is the blood pressure when the heart relaxes between beats.

A *manometer* is used to measure blood pressure. An indication of low, normal and high readings is given in the diagram. The figures are a rough guide and are usually considered in conjunction with other factors.

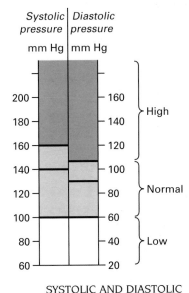

SYSTOLIC AND DIASTOLIC BLOOD PRESSURE

The lymphatic system

This is a secondary circulation intertwined with the blood circulation. The basic material of the lymphatic system in the *lymph* which is a pale yellow fluid similar in composition to interstitial fluid. It gives nourishment to the tissue cells and in return takes away their waste products. The liquid is drained off by tiny lymphatic vessels which join together to form larger lymph vessels and, as these lymph vessels convey lymph towards the heart, they are supplied with valves in much the same way as veins. Along their course towards the heart there are receiving or reservoir areas known as *lymph nodes*. They vary in size from a pin head to a small almond. The purpose of these lymph nodes is to filter the lymph as it passes through and, in this way, to help prevent infection passing into the blood stream and to add *lymphocytes* to the lymph.

Eventually all lymph passes into two principal lymph vessels, the *thoracic duct* and the right *lymphatic duct*, which open into the blood stream at the junctions of the right and left internal, jugular and subclavian veins where it becomes part of the general systemic circulation again.

There are approximately 100 of these lymphatic nodes scattered throughout the body along the line of the lymphatic vessels. The most common superficial ones are the *inguinals* in the groin, the nodes in the *popliteal fossa* (depression behind the knee), the *supratrochlea* in the crutch of the elbow, the *axillary glands* in the armpit, the *supraclavicular glands*, the *submandibular glands* underneath the mandible and the *cervical* and *occipital glands*. These superficial glands are the ones which swell when an infection is present in that part of the body.

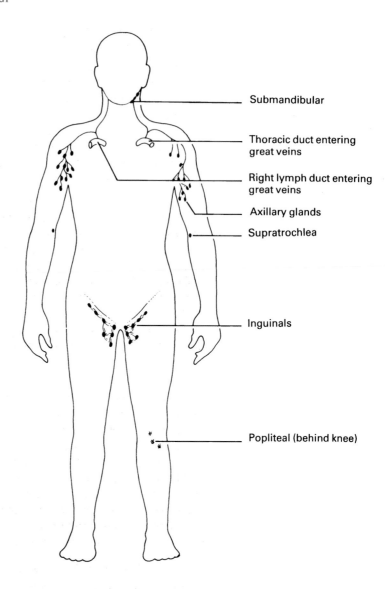

THE LYMPH NODES

Conditions, deficiencies and diseases of the vascular system

Anaemia   This is probably the most common blood complaint. It is a loss of normal balance between the productive and destructive blood processes. This can be due to a drop in the blood volume after a haemorrhage, or a drop in the number of red blood cells, or in the amount of haemoglobin, or a combination of any two or more of these factors.

There are many forms of anaemia but we are primarily concerned with two categories:

- *simple anaemia* In simple anaemia there are two direct causative factors. The first is a marked nutritional deficiency of iron, frequently seen in the premature infant, the growing child, and the pregnant

48

woman. The second causative factor is chronic blood loss, for example during menstruation or as a result of an accident.

- *pernicious anaemia* One of the characteristics of pernicious anaemia is the presence of giant red cells (*macrocytes*), each cell appearing to be overloaded with haemoglobin, whilst the total red cells count is decreased. As recently as 1925 this disease was invariably fatal, but today the life expectancy of the properly treated patient is about the same as that of the general population. Basically, pernicious anaemia results from failure of red blood cells to develop and mature normally.

Whilst a decreased number of red blood cells is indicative of anaemia, a continuously increasing number of white blood cells can be indicative of *leukaemia*. Reference has already been made to the fact that white blood cells increase in number by mitosis in the presence of the necessary stimuli such as an infection and the normal 8000 per cubic millimetre of blood can increase to as many as 60 000 in a case of severe pneumonia. However, when the condition is cured, the mitosing or dividing ceases and the white blood count returns to normal. In leukaemia the leucocytes and/or lymphocytes do not remain at the normal number but gradually increase.

Varicose veins

A network of veins serves to drain the capillary beds and body tissue of 'used' blood, and returns this blood to the heart. Venous flow is assisted in its return to the heart by the rhythmic suction action of breathing, muscular contraction in the extremities and the valves located in the veins. Gravity assists the venous blood from the neck and head to return to the heart, but venous flow from the legs is against the pull of gravity and, for most of the day, has to run uphill. The valves in the veins prevent back flow and when some of these valves become impaired or cease to function the veins become permanently dilated. There are many causes of varicose veins, including:

- *congenital factors* – varicosity appears to run in families
- *environmental factors* – people whose work necessitates their standing still for long periods of time are at particular risk.

Varicose veins are also, quite often, a complication of pregnancy and obesity.

Haemophilia

This is the best known of the bleeding diseases. It is a hereditary disease – the victim is usually male and the disease is passed on by the mother, who is the so-called carrier. It is a disease in which there is a deficiency in the clotting of the blood.

Blue baby

This is a baby born with a congenital structural defect of the heart which results in a constant recirculation of some of the venous blood without its prior passage through the lungs to pick up oxygen. The degree of blueness is, at least in part, dependent on the size of the hole through which the venous blood passes.

Arteriosclerosis and atherosclerosis These two conditions are often confused because of the similarity in many of the symptoms. Simply:

- *Arteriosclerosis* is hardening of the arterial walls brought about mainly by degenerative changes which increase in frequency with age.
- *Atherosclerosis* is a build-up of cholesterol on the inside of the artery which reduces the size of the bore.

Blood transfusions

The transfer of blood to a recipient from a donor is one of the very widely used procedures in medical treatments – making up deficiencies caused by severe haemorrhage and, in some cases, when the blood volume is normal, a transfusion is used in order to replace a deficiency in one of the constituents of the blood.

The first record we have of a transfusion was of one performed between two dogs by a Richard Lower in England in 1665. Soon after this it was tried in France but the results on humans were so disastrous that the French passed a law forbidding transfusions. It was not until the early twentieth century, when Karl Landsteiner completed his blood grouping, that progress was made in the field of human transfusions. Because, at that time, they had no means of keeping the blood fresh, only direct transfusions were possible. In 1914 Louis Agote of Argentina found that sodium citrate could be used for this purpose and the discovery was used extensively in the First World War. Since that time new methods have been found for obtaining and keeping blood for use at some future time and blood banks have become an accepted part of our medical system.

GLOSSARY

Angiology	the science dealing with blood vessels and lymphatics
Cholesterol	a constituent of all animal fats and oils, insoluble in water. Its presence on the inside walls of blood vessels contributes to hypertension and other cardio-vascular conditions.
Coronary	relating to the heart
Diastolic pressure	the pressure measured during the relaxing phase of the cardiac cycle
Electrocardiogram (ECG)	a graphic record of heart activity made on an instrument known as an electro-cardiograph
Haemorrhoids (Piles)	dilated veins in the rectum and anus, described as internal or external depending on their position

Hypertension	high blood pressure
Hypotension	low blood pressure
Phlebitis	an inflammation of the vein walls, most common in the legs. It may lead to thrombo-phlebitis, a complication caused by an obstructing blood clot.
Systolic pressure	the pressure measured during the contraction phase of the cardiac cycle
Thrombus	a clot of blood found within the heart or blood vessels
Tricuspid and Mitral	valves of the heart

6 The Neurological System

The neurological (or nervous) system transmits and receives messages to and from the brain and all parts of the body. There are two main divisions:

- the *central nervous system*, also known as the cerebrospinal system because it consists of the brain and the spinal cord

- the *autonomic nervous system*, which includes the sympathetic system and the parasympathetic system.

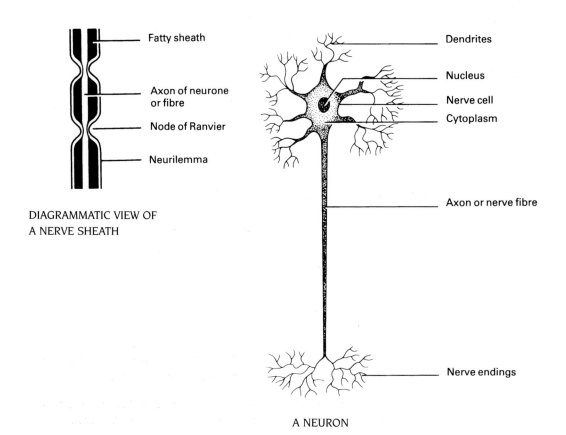

Fatty sheath

Axon of neurone or fibre

Node of Ranvier

Neurilemma

DIAGRAMMATIC VIEW OF
A NERVE SHEATH

Dendrites

Nucleus

Nerve cell

Cytoplasm

Axon or nerve fibre

Nerve endings

A NEURON

The basis of the nervous system is the *nerve cell* or *neuron*. This consists of a nerve cell body with its receiving processes, the *dendrites*, and its transmitting process, the *axon* and its *nerve endings*. White nerve fibres are *medullated*, that is they are enclosed in a sheath of *myelin*. Grey nerve fibres are non-medullated, that is, they have no myelin.

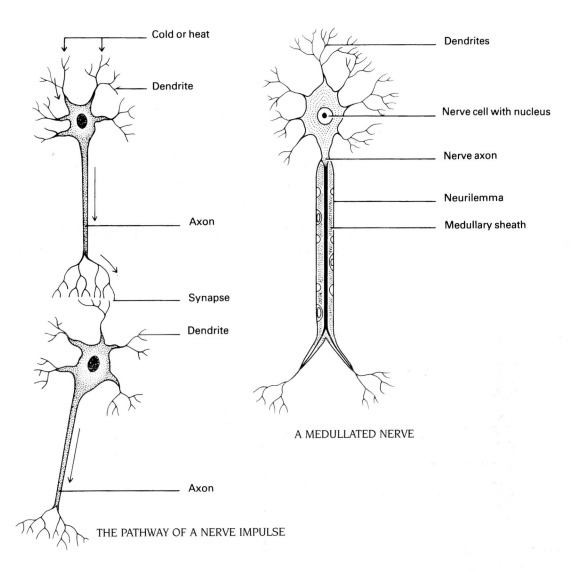

THE PATHWAY OF A NERVE IMPULSE

A MEDULLATED NERVE

The central nervous system

The brain The brain is at the centre of the central nervous system. It is well protected from the outside by the hard bone structure of the skull. Inside, the brain is protected by three membranes, the *meninges*:

- the outer layer, the *dura mater* (strong or hard mother), which is constructed of strong fibrous tissue anchored to the skull

- the middle layer, the *arachnoid*, which is more delicate than the dura mater and is not anchored to the skull. Beneath it is a large reservoir of cerebral spinal fluid which surrounds the brain and on which it rests

- inner layer, the *pia mater* (soft mother), which is in contact with the grey matter of the brain itself and dips deep down between the brain convolutions.

The adult human brain weighs rather more than 1360 g and is so full of water that it tends to slump rather like a blancmange if placed without the support of a firm surface. It is estimated that it has 12 billion neurons or nerve cells.

When we speak of the brain we are really considering three quite different structures:

- the *cerebrum*
- the *cerebellum*
- the *medulla oblongata*.

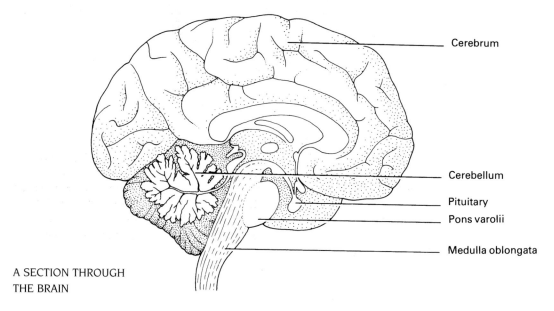

Cerebrum

Cerebellum

Pituitary

Pons varolii

Medulla oblongata

A SECTION THROUGH THE BRAIN

The cerebrum

The cerebrum consists of two symmetrical hemispheres. The outer layer of the cerebrum is known as the *cortex* and this is arranged in convolutions, that is deep irregularly shaped fissures or indentations. This is the grey matter of the brain. Underneath the cortex lies nerve fibre or white matter. The function of the cerebrum is to control voluntary movement and to receive and interpret conscious sensations. It is the seat of the higher functions such as the senses, memory, reasoning, intelligence and moral sense.

The cerebellum

The cerebellum is much smaller in size and lies below and behind the cerebrum. It too has grey matter under which is white matter. Its function is to control muscular co-ordination and balance.

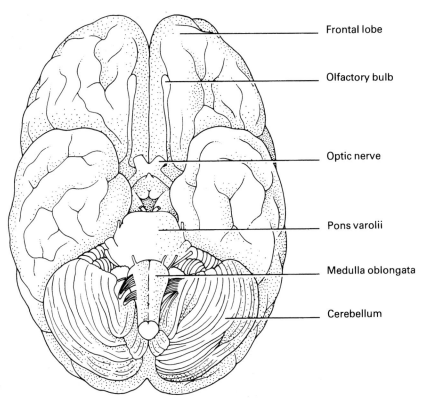

THE BRAIN VIEWED FROM BELOW

Labels: Frontal lobe, Olfactory bulb, Optic nerve, Pons varolii, Medulla oblongata, Cerebellum

The medulla oblongata

The medulla oblongata is about 3 cm long, tapering from its greatest width of 2 cm and connecting the rest of the brain with the spinal cord with which it is continuous. It is made up of interspersed white and grey matter. The medulla oblongata not only acts as the link between the brain and the central nervous system of the body but it is also the centre of those parts of the autonomic nervous system which control the heart, lungs, processes of digestion, etc.

Other parts of the brain include:

- the *pons varoli*
- the *pituitary gland*
- the *hypothalamus*.

The *pons varoli*

The *pons varoli* is a bridge of nerve fibres linking the right and left hemispheres and also the cerebellum with the cerebrum above and the medulla oblongata below. All impulses which pass between the brain and the spinal cord traverse the *pons varoli*.

The pituitary gland

The pituitary gland (or hypophysis) is a small gland about the size of a pea and lies in the pituitary fossa in the base of the skull. Its function is dealt with in Chapter 10, the Endocrine System.

55

The hypothalamus

The hypothalamus is situated in the area of the floor of the third ventricle of the brain and it exercises an influence over the autonomic nervous system. It contains the heat regulating centre and is generally believed to be involved with appetite.

The spinal cord The spinal cord, which is continuous with the medulla oblongata, extends downwards through the vertebrae of the spinal column. The cord itself is cylindrical in shape with an outer covering of supporting cells and blood vessels and an inner egg-shaped core of *nerve fibres*. It extends through four-fifths of the spinal column and is about 45 cm in length.

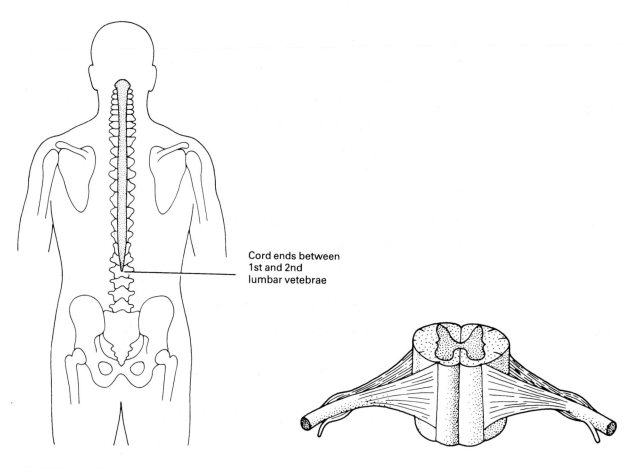

Cord ends between 1st and 2nd lumbar vetebrae

THE POSITION OF THE SPINAL CORD

A SECTION THROUGH THE SPINAL CORD

Nerves There are 12 pairs of *cranial nerves* given off from the base of the brain; 31 other pairs branch off the spinal cord throughout its length. These extend to every part of the body. Nerves that extend upwards through the spinal cord to the brain pass through the medulla oblongata where they cross – thus the left-hand side of the brain controls the right-hand side of the body, whilst the right-hand side of the brain controls the left-hand side of the body. Nerves of the central nervous system fall into three categories:

- *motor* or *efferent nerves*, whose primary function is to control the movement of muscles
- *sensory* or *afferent nerves*, which carry impulses from the sensory nerve endings to the spinal column and the brain
- *mixed nerves*, which consist of both motor and sensory fibres.

Cranial nerves

Name	Type	Function	Number
Abducent	Motor	Supplies lateral rectus muscles of eyes	6
Auditory	Sensory	Sense of hearing, maintenance of balance, equilibrium	8
Facial	Mixed	Sense of taste from tongue and impulses to muscles of facial expression	7
Glosso-pharyngeal	Mixed	Sensations from tongue, impulses to muscles of pharynx	9
Hypoglossal	Motor	Supplies tongue muscles	12
Oculomotor	Motor	Supplies muscles operating eyes	3
Olfactory	Sensory	Sense of smell	1
Optic	Sensory	Sense of sight	2
Trochlear	Motor	Supplies superior oblique muscles of eyes	4
Trigeminal	Mixed	Receiving pain, heat, pressure and stimulating muscles of mastication	5
Spinal accessory	Motor	To sterno-cleido mastoid and trapezius muscles	11
Vagus	Mixed	Sensory, motor, digestive and respiratory organs	10

Spinal nerves

The 31 pairs of spinal nerves comprise:

- 8 pairs of cervical nerves
- 12 pairs of thoracic nerves
- 5 pairs of lumbar nerves
- 5 pairs of sacral nerves
- 1 pair of coccygeal nerves.

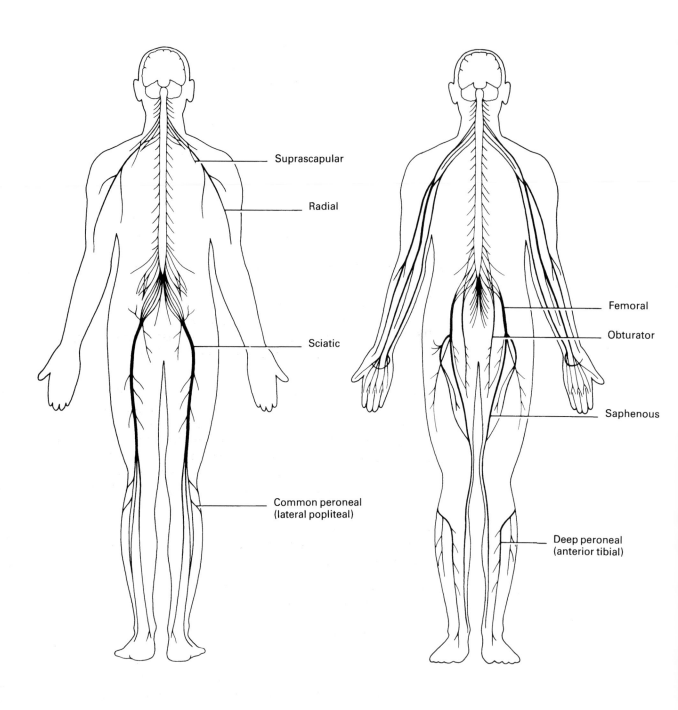

Suprascapular

Radial

Sciatic

Common peroneal
(lateral popliteal)

Femoral

Obturator

Saphenous

Deep peroneal
(anterior tibial)

NERVES (POSTERIOR BODY)

NERVES (ANTERIOR BODY)

The autonomic nervous system

This controls all body structures over which we have no voluntary control. It is divided into two separate parts:

- the *sympathetic system*
- the *parasympathetic system*.

The sympathetic system

The sympathetic system comprises a gangliated cord which runs on either side of the front of the vertebral column. The principal plexuses of this system are:

- the *cardiac plexus*, which supplies all the thoracic viscera and the thoracic vessels
- the *coeliac* or *solar plexus*, which supplies all the abdominal viscera
- the *hypogastric plexus*, which supplies the pelvic organs.

The parasympathetic system

The parasympathetic nervous system consists mainly of the *vagus nerve* which gives off branches to the organs of the thorax and abdomen, but also includes branches from other cranial nerves, mainly the third, seventh and ninth as well as nerves in the sacral region of the spinal column.

All the internal organs therefore have a double nerve supply from the sympathetic and parasympathetic systems and their effect is opposite – simply, a sympathetic nerve has the effect of increasing body activity and speeds it up, whereas the parasympathetic, on the contrary, slows down body activity.

The sympathetic fibres increase the heart rate, raise the blood pressure, mobilise glucose, stimulate the secretion of sweat. The parasympathetic fibres slow the heart, lower the blood pressure and decrease the secretion of sweat. It has been maintained that the sympathetic system provides for today's work and that its action increases when involved with physical activity. The parasympathetic, on the other hand, looks after tomorrow, being mainly concerned with changes which take place during rest.

The sympathetic nerves are stimulated by strong emotions such as anger and excitement. In fact it is because of this effect of the emotions that they are called sympathetic.

The *adrenal* is one of the glands which they stimulate and the liberation of *adrenalin* is one of the body's responses to anger. In some people, the parasympathetic nerves are the stronger and hold the balance in the body; such people generally have a placid disposition, good digestion and are not very easily disturbed. These are known as *vagotonic* types. In other people, the sympathetic nerves are the stronger and these people are more emotional, less stable and their digestion is more readily disturbed. These are known as *sympatheticotonic* types.

Another function of the autonomic nervous system is related to the reflex nervous action. This is an involuntary reaction to a stimulation, for example, taking the fingers away quickly from a hot surface, the recovery of balance to prevent a fall, and so on. It is also within this system that a reflex action is *conditioned*. For example, the normal reflex action when handed a very hot plate would be to drop it, but as this action would carry with it certain distinct disadvantages, like loss of the meal that was on the plate or the work involved with clearing up afterwards, the plate – instead of being dropped – is quickly put down. That is a reflex action which has been conditioned by other considerations.

Conditions and diseases of the neurological system

Neuritis   This takes in a wide group of disturbances which affect the peripheral nerves after they leave the spinal cord. Some of the disturbances are due to infection, others to compression of the nerves. Probably the biggest single factor is the build-up of urea and lactic acid at a point, or points, of the nerve's course, which affects the nerve's sheathing.

Bell's Palsy (Facial paralysis)   This is a neuritis of the facial nerve usually caused by infection and compression of the swollen nerve as it passes through a tiny opening in the skull below the ear in its course to the muscles of the face.

Neuralgia   This is a painful condition in a nerve due to irritation, inflammation or exposure.

Parkinson's Disease   Otherwise known as *Paralysis Agitans*, this is an extremely common illness beginning in middle life, deriving from disease of the basal ganglia. The disease is slowly progressive but, as it does not affect the brain, intelligence is unaffected. The chief symptoms of this illness are tremor, rigidity and slowness of movement.

Sciatica   This is inflammation of the great sciatic nerve, the longest single nerve in the body. This is often a form of rheumatic neuritis but it can also be caused by compression, an arthritic spur or a prolapsed intravertebral disc.

GLOSSARY

Brachial neuritis	a condition similar to sciatica but in the arm
Ganglia	a group of nerve cell bodies usually located outside the brain and spinal cord

Plexus   a network of interlacing nerves

Spasticity   a stage of sustained contraction of a muscle associated with an exaggeration of deep reflexes

Synapse   the region of communication between neurons; the point at which an impulse passes from an axon of one neuron to a dendrite of the cell body of another

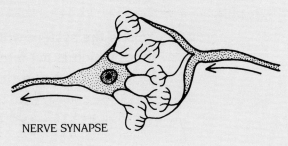

NERVE SYNAPSE

7 The Digestive System

This is the system which is responsible for changing the food, which is *put into* the body, into substances suitable for absorption and therefore *usable by* the body.

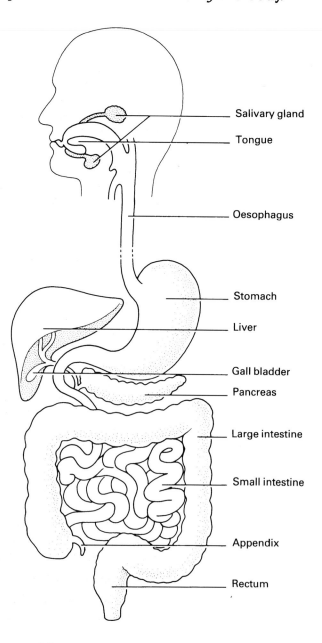

Salivary gland

Tongue

Oesophagus

Stomach

Liver

Gall bladder

Pancreas

Large intestine

Small intestine

Appendix

Rectum

THE DIGESTIVE SYSTEM

As the health and efficient working of the body must depend, to a very large extent, on the food which is put into it and the treatment which the food receives, it is necessary to have at least a basic understanding of the processes involved and some of the ways in which they may go wrong. The body needs material for growth, repair, heat and energy and these materials are supplied by the foods we eat. It is the digestive system which produces the chemical and other changes which make it possible for the food to perform functions necessary to maintain life.

Organs of the digestive tract

The digestive tract, or alimentary canal, is more than 10 m long. It is continuous, starting at the *mouth*, passing through the *pharynx*, the *oesophagus*, the *stomach*, the *small* and *large intestine* and ending with the *rectum* and the *anus*. Associated with it are accessory organs: the *tongue*, *teeth*, *salivary glands*, *liver* and *pancreas*.

Teeth

There are 32 permanent teeth; working from the front backwards on each side of the jaw, there are *two incisors*, *one canine* or eye tooth, *two premolars* or bicuspids and *three molars*.

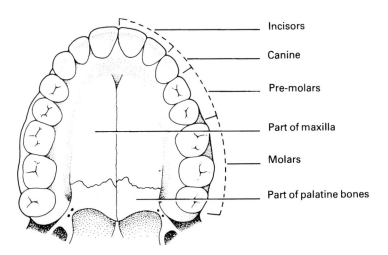

THE TEETH AND BONY PALATE

Incisors

Canine

Pre-molars

Part of maxilla

Molars

Part of palatine bones

The tongue

The tongue consists of striated voluntary muscle and is attached mainly to the mandible and hyoid bones. The upper surface of the tongue is covered with papillae. There are three types of papillae:

- the *filliform papillae*, found chiefly on the dorsum of the tongue
- the *fungiform papillae*, found mainly on the sides and tip of the tongue

- the *vallate papillae*, lying in a V-formation at the back of the tongue. Taste buds are resident in the walls of the vallate papillae.

Salivary glands

There are three pairs of salivary glands:

- the *parotid glands* in front of and below the ears
- the *sublingual glands* below the tongue
- the *submandibular glands* below the mandible.

The salivary glands produce secretions containing the enzyme, *ptyalin*, which helps in the digestion of cooked starches.

The pharynx

From the mouth the food passes into the pharynx which is a muscular tube that has seven openings into it. These are the *mouth*, the *oesophagus, the larynx, two posterior apertures of the nose* and *two auditory (Eustachian) tubes from the ear.*

The oesophagus

From the pharynx the food passes into the oesophagus which is a muscular tube lined with mucous membrane and covered with fibrous tissue.

The stomach

From the oesophagus the food passes into the stomach which is a muscular sac, its size and shape varying with its contents and muscular tone. The stomach presents two curvatures, the *greater* and the *lesser curvature* and is divided into three parts – the *cardiac portion*, the *body* and the *pyloric*. The openings into the stomach are guarded by circular bands of muscle, the *cardiac sphincter muscle* at one end and the *pyloric sphincter* muscle at the other.

The stomach has three coats or coverings, the outer coat of *serous membrane*, the *middle muscular coat* and the *inner mucous membrane*. This mucous membrane is arranged in folds, or *rugae*, which disappear when the stomach is distended. The membrane is lined with glands which produce gastric juice. This contains the enzymes *pepsin* (responsible for protein digestion) and *rennin* (responsible for the curdling of milk) and also hydrochloric acid.

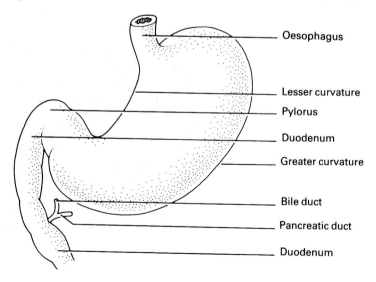

Oesophagus

Lesser curvature

Pylorus

Duodenum

Greater curvature

Bile duct

Pancreatic duct

Duodenum

THE STOMACH (ANTERIOR VIEW)

The small intestine　From the stomach the food passes into the smaller intestine, the first part of this being the *duodenum* which is about 25 cm long and shaped like a letter 'C'. The remainder of the small intestine consists of the *jejunum* which is about 2.5 m long and the *ileum* which is about 3.5 m long. The inner coat of the small intestine is comprised of mucous membrane arranged in folds known as *valvulae conniventes* and, unlike the rugae of the stomach, these folds do not disappear with the distension of the intestines.

The mucous membrane is covered with minute fingerlike projections known as *villi*; each villus contains a lacteal for the absorption of fat and a capillary loop for the absorption of sugar and protein. This mucous membrane also contains intestinal glands which produce a secretion known as *succus entericus* which contains enzymes for the digestion of protein and sugars. The mucous membrane is studded with lymphatic nodules and, in the latter part of the small intestine, that is in the ileum, groups of these nodules are found and are known as Peyer's *patches*, their function being to fight infection. The small intestine then merges with the large intestine which though wider than the small intestine is much shorter, about 1.5 m long.

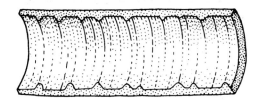

SECTION OF SMALL INTESTINE
(SHOWING PUCKERED LINING OF
VALVULAE CONNIVENTES)

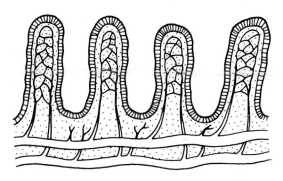

ENLARGED SECTION OF SMALL INTESTINE WALL
(SHOWING VILLI)

The large intestine　The large intestine can be divided into nine parts; it starts with the *caecum* into which the ileum opens. The opening is guarded by the *ileo-caecal valve* which allows onflow but prevents backflow of intestinal contents. The *vermiform appendix* is attached to the blind end of the caecum and is about 7.5 cm long. The *ascending colon* passes upwards from the caecum along the right side of the abdomen and bends sharply to the left at the *right* or *hepatic flexure* to become the *transverse colon*. This passes across the abdominal cavity and turns sharply downwards at the *left* or *splenic flexure* to continue as the *descending colon*. This goes down the left side of the abdomen to the *sigmoid flexure* in the pelvic cavity and the *rectum*. The rectum is about 13 cm long with two sphincter muscles at the exit, or *anus*.

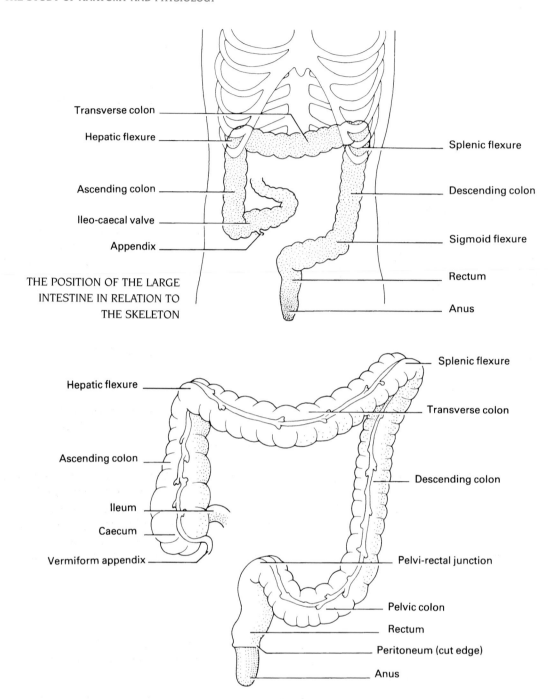

Transverse colon

Hepatic flexure

Splenic flexure

Ascending colon

Descending colon

Ileo-caecal valve

Sigmoid flexure

Appendix

Rectum

THE POSITION OF THE LARGE
INTESTINE IN RELATION TO
THE SKELETON

Anus

Hepatic flexure

Splenic flexure

Transverse colon

Ascending colon

Descending colon

Ileum

Caecum

Vermiform appendix

Pelvi-rectal junction

Pelvic colon

Rectum

Peritoneum (cut edge)

Anus

THE LARGE INTESTINE

The liver The liver is situated on the right-hand side of the body just below the diaphragm. This is really a gland and is the largest gland in the body. It measures about 25–30 cm across and 15–18 cm from back to front; it weighs approximately 1.5 kg. It is divided into two lobes – the large right lobe and the smaller left lobe. The right lobe is subdivided into the *quadrate* and *caudate* lobes. The liver has many functions and one of these is the formation and storage of bile – of which it produces up to 1 litre in a day. This passes to the *gall bladder* which is a muscular, pear-

66

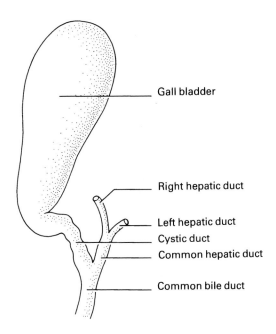

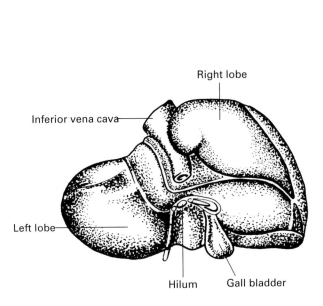

THE LIVER (SEEN FROM BEHIND)

THE GALL BLADDER AND ITS DUCTS

shaped sac about 7.5 cm long. Its function is to store bile and to concentrate it by eight to ten times; when required, the bile passes out of the gall bladder into the duodenum.

The pancreas The pancreas is a cream-coloured gland, 15–20 cm long and about 4 cm wide. It is divided into the head, neck, body and tail. A duct, running the length of the organ, collects pancreatic juice and passes it to the duodenum at the same point that the common bile duct passes in bile. The *islets of Langerhans* are specialised cells of the pancreas which produce *insulin*. This is passed into the general circulation and controls carbohydrate metabolism.

Some notes on digestion

Digestive juices contain *enzymes* which break down food. Enzymes are proteins which speed up chemical reactions – they are biological catalysts.

During the digestive process, large particles of protein, carbohydrate and fat are reduced in size and converted into simpler substances enabling them to be absorbed through the walls of the digestive tract into the blood stream.

Proteins are broken down to *peptones* and *polypeptides* and finally *amino acids*. Large particles of carbohydrates (starches or polysaccharides) are reduced to *disaccharides* which, in turn, are reduced to *monosaccharides*. Fats are split into their component parts, *fatty acids* and *glycerol*.

It should be noted that with one or two exceptions there is no absorption of food elements until they reach the intestine, where fatty

67

acids and glycerol pass into the lacteals of the villi and amino acids into the capillary blood vessels. Fatty products are conveyed to the lymphatic system and enter the systemic circulation via the *thoracic duct*. Amino acids and simple sugars are carried by the portal vein to the liver.

The movement of food along the digestive tract is made possible by wavelike, muscular contractions known as *peristalsis*. The action is from the outside of the digestive tubes inwards and downwards, so that the food is forced further along the tube.

The stomach, being a muscularly controlled sac, is always on the move and might be compared with an old fashioned butter churn where the food is pushed around until it is well and truly mixed with gastric juice, a mixture of enzymes in hydrochloric acid.

As we have already seen, the stomach has a pyloric valve at the point where it merges into the small intestine. The function of this valve is to control the release of the partially digested food material into the small intestine. Watery foods, such as soup, leave the stomach quite quickly, whilst fats remain considerably longer. An ordinary mixed diet meal is emptied from the stomach in 3–5 hours.

It has already been seen that the liver manufactures and stores bile but it has a variety of other functions. It is a powerful detoxifying organ, breaking down many kinds of toxic molecules and rendering them harmless. It is a storage organ for some vitamins and digested carbohydrate in the form of glycogen, which it releases to sustain blood sugar levels. It manufactures enzymes, cholesterol, proteins, vitamin A from carotene, blood coagulation factors and other substances.

Bile is a complex fluid containing, amongst other things, bile salts and bile pigments. The pigments are derived from the disintegration of red blood cells and give the yellow brown colour of the faeces which are excreted. The bile salts are reabsorbed and reused; they promote efficient digestion of fats by a detergent action which gives very fine emulsification of fatty materials.

Conditions and diseases of the digestive system

Appendicitis
This is an acute inflammation of the vermiform appendix. A distended, inflamed appendix may rupture and produce toxic materials, which can cause peritonitis, an acute inflammation of the abdomen.

Cirrhosis of the liver
There are several types of cirrhosis of the liver but *portal cirrhosis* is, by far, the most common. This is also referred to as gin drinker's liver, or alcoholic liver. It is usually caused by exposure to poison, which can include such substances as carbon tetrachloride and phosphorus, but by far the most common cause is the ingestion of alcohol. This makes the liver leathery and produces nodules on its normally smooth surface – varying in size from a pin head to a bean – which give it a hobnailed appearance.

Jaundice Jaundice is normally evidenced by the yellowness of the skin caused by an excess of bile pigments in the circulatory system. It may occur when the outflow of the bile has been blocked and when the liver surface itself is inflamed. When the small bile duct within the liver becomes obstructed a large portion of the bile which is produced by the liver is absorbed directly into the blood stream, as it cannot flow normally out of the bile duct into the duodenum.

Heartburn (Pyrosis) This is a common symptom of gastric distress consisting of a burning sensation which extends up into the oesophagus and quite often into the throat and is accompanied by a sour belch.

8 The Respiratory System

The respiratory system is responsible for taking in oxygen and giving off carbon dioxide and some water. The process of taking in air into the body is *inspiration* and getting rid of air from the body is *expiration*.

An average adult breathes something like 13 650 litres of air a day. This is not only the body's largest intake of any substance but also the most vital. It is possible to live without food for many days, without water for a few days but without air only for a very few minutes.

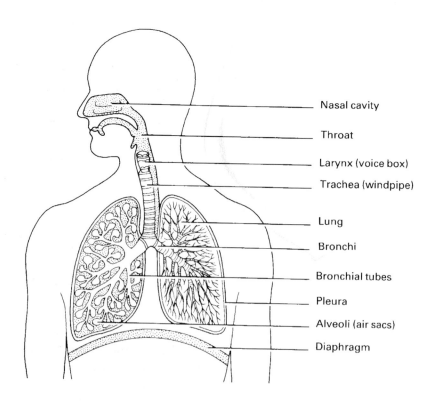

THE RESPIRATORY SYSTEM

Nasal cavity

Throat

Larynx (voice box)

Trachea (windpipe)

Lung

Bronchi

Bronchial tubes

Pleura

Alveoli (air sacs)

Diaphragm

70

Organs of the respiratory system

The respiratory system is divided into:

- the *upper respiratory tract*, which includes the nose, mouth, throat, larynx and sinus cavities in the head
- the *lower respiratory tract*, which includes the trachea (windpipe), bronchi, diaphragm and lungs.

Air brought in through the nose is filtered and warmed before passing down to the lungs.

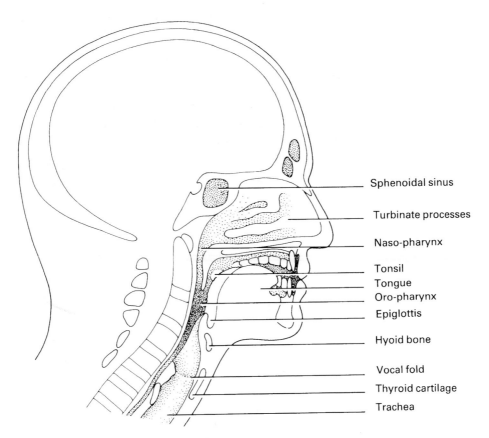

Sphenoidal sinus

Turbinate processes

Naso-pharynx

Tonsil
Tongue
Oro-pharynx
Epiglottis

Hyoid bone

Vocal fold
Thyroid cartilage
Trachea

THE UPPER RESPIRATORY TRACT

The two lungs are the principal organs of the respiratory system and are situated in the upper part of the thoracic cage. They are inert organs, that is they do not work by themselves but function by a variation of atmospheric pressure which is achieved by a muscular wall known as the *diaphragm*.

The diaphragm The contraction and relaxation of the diaphragm result in an alteration in the volume of the thorax, and therefore an alteration of atmospheric pressure within the lungs themselves.

The diaphragm when relaxed is a flattened dome shape pointing upwards to the lungs. When it contracts, it flattens, pulls down the thorax, increases the volume of the thorax, and thus decreases the

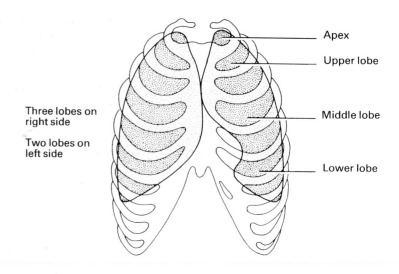

Apex

Upper lobe

Three lobes on
right side

Two lobes on
left side

Middle lobe

Lower lobe

THE POSITION OF THE LUNGS
WITHIN THE THORAX

atmospheric pressure in the lungs. This causes air to rush in –
inspiration. When the diaphragm relaxes, the thorax is pushed up, the
volume decreases and the atmospheric pressure increases, and air
rushes out of the lungs – *expiration*. The inspired air, which contains
oxygen, passes down into the billions of minute air chambers or air
cells known as *alveoli* which have very thin walls. Around these walls are
the capillaries of the pulmonary system. It is at this point that the fresh
air gives off its oxygen to the blood and takes carbon dioxide from the
blood which is then expelled with the expired air.

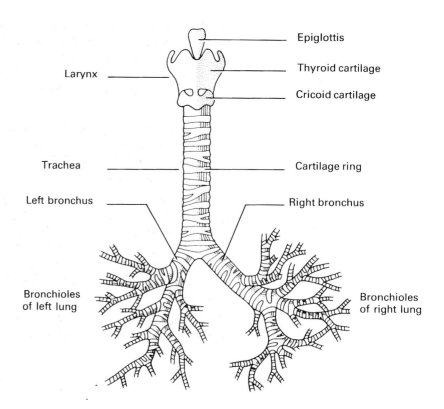

Epiglottis

Thyroid cartilage

Larynx

Cricoid cartilage

Trachea

Cartilage ring

Left bronchus

Right bronchus

Bronchioles
of left lung

Bronchioles
of right lung

THE LOWER RESPIRATORY TRACT

The trachea The trachea (or windpipe) measures about 11.5 cm in length and is approximately 2.5 cm in diameter. It has rings of cartilage to prevent it collapsing. It passes through the neck in front of the oesophagus branching into two bronchi – the right bronchus being 2.5 cm long and the left bronchus 5 cm long. The bronchi branch into smaller and smaller tubes ending in the bronchioles which have no cartilage in their walls and have clusters of the thin-walled air sacs – alveoli.

The lungs The lungs are greyish in colour and are spongy in appearance. The right lung has three lobes – upper, middle and lower, and the left lung has two lobes – upper and lower.

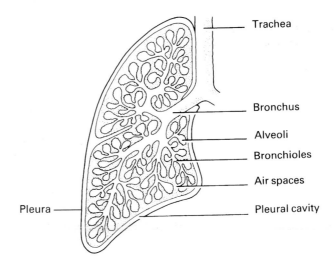

- Trachea
- Bronchus
- Alveoli
- Bronchioles
- Air spaces
- Pleural cavity

Pleura

A SECTION OF THE LUNG

The *pleura* is the serous membrane which covers the lungs. The *visceral layer* is in close contact with the lung tissue and the *parietal layer* lines the chest wall. Between these layers is the *pleural cavity*. In health it is a natural cavity because the two membranes are fluid lubricated on their opposing surfaces and slide easily over each other as the lungs expand and contract.

Air going into the lungs follows the same throat passageway as food for a short distance, but there is an ingenious trapdoor called the *epiglottis* which permits the passage of air to the lungs but closes it when food or liquids are swallowed.

During normal quiet breathing about 0.5 litres of air flow in and out of the lungs. This is known as *tidal air*. If inhalation is continued at the end of ordinary breathing, an additional 1.5 litres of *complemental air* can be forced into the lungs. If exhalation is continued, an extra 1.5 litres of *supplemental air* can be forced out of the lungs. About 1 litre of air remains in the lungs and cannot be expelled – this is known as *residual air*.

The normal rate of inspiration and expiration, the *respiration rate*, is about 16 times a minute in an adult.

Conditions and diseases of the respiratory system

Bronchitis   Bronchitis means inflammation of the bronchi. This occurs when mucus builds up in the airways in excessive amounts and causes coughing. The bronchi may become narrow, making it harder to breathe. It occurs in two forms:

- *acute bronchitis*, which is a short-term illness, usually lasts a week or two, and may result from inhaled materials, such as fog, smoke or chemicals, or may be connected with another condition, such as influenza, measles or whooping cough
- *chronic bronchitis*, which is a long-term illness and may last for months or even years. It is more prevalent in later life and affects about four times as many men as women. It can prove fatal and about 30 000 deaths are recorded annually in the UK from it. People who smoke are at greater risk of chronic bronchitis. It is often linked to *emphysema* (see below).

Emphysema   In emphysema the alveoli of the lungs are gradually destroyed, so sufferers have difficulty absorbing enough oxygen. The bronchi may also become narrow so that it becomes harder to breathe. The most common cause of damage to the alveoli is cigarette smoke.

Like chronic bronchitis, emphysema tends to occur in older people, particularly those who smoke. A small proportion of cases are caused by an inherited problem.

Emphysema and chronic bronchitis often occur together. This is called *chronic obstructive airways disease* (COAD).

Pleurisy   Practically any disease that causes inflammation of the lungs may result in pleurisy. The pleura becomes inflamed and fluids accumulate in the pleural cavity.

Pneumoconiosis   This is a lung condition involving inflammation by minute particles of mineral dusts. It is often called miners' disease or miners' lung due to its prevalence amongst this body of workers. There are, however, a number of other occupations where fine dust is a hazard. Workers who are exposed to a high concentration of silica dust, for example, may develop a variation of the disease known as *pneumosilicosis*. Precautionary measures like the wearing of masks help to reduce the incidence of this disease.

Pulmonary tuberculosis   The disease we know as tuberculosis has been with us for thousands of years. Centuries before Christ it was called *phythisis*, a Greek word meaning wastage or decay. This explains the familiar word for this disease – consumption. It was in 1882 that a German bacteriologist, Robert Koch, discovered that tuberculosis was caused by a long, thin bacterium called *tubercle bacillus*.

GLOSSARY

Asthma   a paroxysmal condition usually due to hypersensitiveness to inhaled or ingested substances, e.g. pollen asthma.

Pneumothorax   collapsed lung – may occur in accidents from bones perforating the chest. Artificial pneumothorax is the introduction of air or other gas into the pleural cavity through a needle in order to produce collapse and immobility of the lung. It is used in the treatment of pulmonary tuberculosis.

Rhinitis   inflammation of the nasal mucous membrane, e.g. acute serous rhinitis – hay fever

9 The Genito-Urinary System

In many anatomical textbooks this system is dealt with as two systems – the *reproductive system* and the *excretive system*. However, as a number of the organs involved are common to both systems the general tendency is to treat them under one heading.

The principal organs involved in the dual system are the *ovaries, fallopian tubes, uterus, testes, urethra, ureter* and the *urinary bladder*.

The female reproductive system

First we have the right and left *ovaries*. These are quite small, about the size of an almond; they consist of masses of very small sacs known as the *ovarian follicles* and each follicle contains an egg – *ovum*. The ovaries have two principal functions:

- to develop the ova and expel one at approximately 28-day intervals during the reproductive life
- to produce hormones (oestrogen and progesterone) which influence secondary sex characteristics and control changes in the uterus during the menstrual cycle.

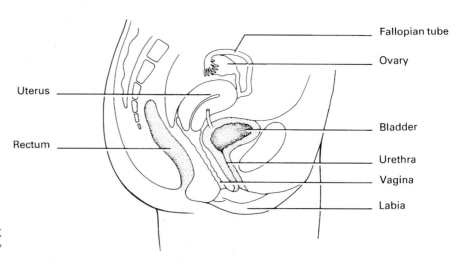

Fallopian tube

Ovary

Uterus

Rectum

Bladder

Urethra

Vagina

Labia

A SECTION OF THE FEMALE
PELVIC CAVITY

The *fallopian tubes*, sometimes referred to as the uterine tubes or *oviducts*, are about 10 cm long and their function is to transport the ova from the ovaries to the uterus.

The *uterus* is a muscular organ approximately pear-shaped, about 7.5 cm long by 5 cm wide and 2.5 cm thick. It is positioned in the centre of the pelvis with the bladder in front and the rectum behind. It is normally divided into three parts – the *fundus*, the broad upper end, the *body*, the central part, and the *cervix* (about 2.5 cm long), the neck which projects into the vagina.

The *vagina* is the muscular canal which connects the above organs to the external body at the point collectively known as the *vulva* which includes the *clitoris* – a small, sensitive organ containing erectile tissue corresponding to the male penis.

The male reproductive system

The male genital organs are fairly simple in comparison to the female genital organs. The principal organs are the *testes*, or testicles, which are the essential male reproductive glands, the *scrotum* which is a pouch-like organ containing the testes, and the *penis* which is suspended in front of the scrotum.

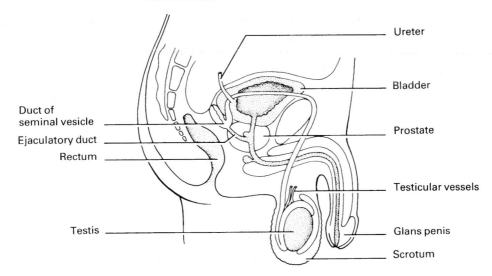

THE MALE GENITAL ORGANS

The excretive system

The kidneys

The kidneys are two bean-shaped organs, approximately 10 cm long, 5 cm wide and 2.5 cm thick. They are positioned against the posterior abdominal wall at the normal waistline, with the right kidney slightly lower than the left.

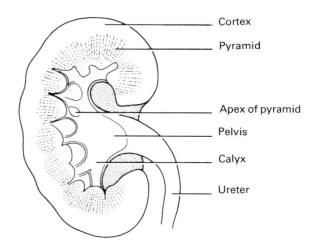

Cortex

Pyramid

Apex of pyramid

Pelvis

Calyx

Ureter

A SECTION OF KIDNEY

The kidneys consist of three principal parts – the *cortex*, or outer layer, which is bright reddish-brown in colour, the *middle portion* or *medulla* which is inside and red striated in colour, and the *pelvis* which is the hollow, inner portion from which the ureters open.

The function of the kidneys is to separate certain waste products from the blood and this renal function helps maintain the blood at a constant level of composition despite the great variation in diet and fluid intake. As blood circulates in the kidneys, a large quantity of water, salts, urea and glucose is filtered into the *capsules of* Bowman and from there into the *convoluted tubules*. From here all the glucose, most of the water and salts and some of the urea are returned to the blood vessels. The remainder passes via the *calyces* into the kidney pelvis as urine. It is estimated that 150–80 litres of fluid are processed by the kidneys each day but only about 1.5 litres of this leaves the body as urine.

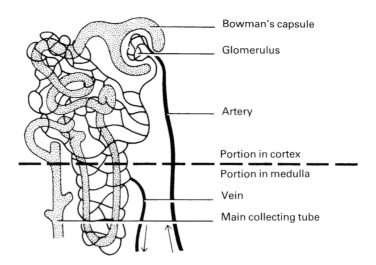

Bowman's capsule

Glomerulus

Artery

Portion in cortex

Portion in medulla

Vein

Main collecting tube

INTERNAL KIDNEY STRUCTURE

The ureters and the bladder The ureters are two fine muscular tubes, 26–30 cm long, which carry the urine from the kidney pelvis to the bladder. This is a very elastic muscular sac lying immediately behind the *symphysis pubis*.

78

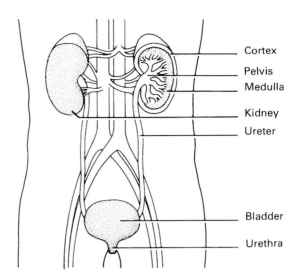

Cortex
Pelvis
Medulla
Kidney
Ureter
Bladder
Urethra

THE EXCRETORY SYSTEM

The urethra The urethra is a narrow muscular tube passing from the bladder to the exterior of the body. The female urethra is 4 cm long and the male urethra 20 cm long.

In the male, the urethra is the common passage for both urine and the semen (reproductive fluid). Also, in the male, it passes through a gland known as the *prostate gland* which is about the size and shape of a chestnut. It surrounds the neck of the bladder and tends to enlarge in later life, interfering with the emptying of the bladder.

Some notes on the functions of the genito-urinary system

Urine composition The average composition of urine is 96 per cent water and 4 per cent solid – 2 per cent urea and 2 per cent salts. The 2 per cent urea compares with 0.04 per cent urea in blood plasma so it will be seen that the concentration has been increased some 50 times by the work of the kidneys. The salts consist mostly of sodium chloride, phosphates and sulphates produced partly from the presence of these salts in protein foods. These salts have either to be reabsorbed or got rid of by the kidneys in sufficient quantities to keep the normal blood balance.

The urine also contains traces of a number of other substances, all of which combine to produce in the urine a reasonable pattern of the state of the body itself. Its analysis indicates a number of physiological states including the amount of alcohol in the body, whether a female is pregnant or not and whether a person has diabetes.

Reproduction It is estimated that, at birth, there are some 30 000 ova or eggs in a female child. No fresh ova are formed after birth but – during the reproductive female life – that is, commencing between 10 and 16 years of age and concluding between 45 and 55 years of age – these ova develop within the follicles or sacs in which they are embedded. They come progressively nearer to the surface of the ovary where they mature and increase in size. About every 28 days, one of these follicles bursts and the ovum it contains, together with the fluid surrounding it, is expelled into the fallopian tubes and thence into the uterus where it may or may not be fertilised. If the ovum is fertilised by a male reproductive cell, or *spermatozoon*, it then attaches itself to the uterine wall and develops there. If the ovum does not become fertilised within a few days it is cast off and the process termed *menstruation* is initiated.

The spermatozoa which are responsible for fertilisation are contained in a substance known as *seminal fluid*. An average ejection of seminal fluid contains several hundred million of these mobile sperm which look rather like miniature elongated tadpoles, about 0.05 mm in length. Each one consists of a headpiece, a middle piece and a long whiplike tail piece. It is this vigorous tail piece or lashing tail which gives the spermatozoon its mobility.

The single fertilised ovum soon becomes many cells which develop in a bag of membranes and soon fill the uterine cavity. At one part of this sac – the point where the ovum first embedded itself in the uterine wall, the *placenta* or afterbirth develops. The umbilical cord contains blood vessels and runs from the navel of the foetus to the placenta. The placenta receives the mother's blood from the wall of the uterus and the infant's blood via the umbilical cord so that, at no stage, does the mother's blood pass directly into the child. It is through the placenta that the child's blood is able to absorb food, oxygen and water from the mother and, in turn, give off its waste products.

The skin The skin is, of course, an organ very closely connected with the excretal system but – as it is a multi-purpose organ – it is dealt with in Chapter 11.

Conditions and diseases of the genito-urinary system

Cervicitis This is an infection of the *cervix* (the neck of the uterus), and is reasonably common. It may be due to gonorrhoea, syphilis or a specific infection.

Cystitis Cystitis is inflammation of the bladder, a condition especially common in women. This is due to the fact that the urethra in women is very short and is a pathway to invasion by infecting organisms.

Kidney stones Stones in the kidney are quite common and precipitate out of the urine, which is a complex solution of many substances. Surgical operations for the removal of stones have a very long history. The Greek doctor, Hippocrates, admonished fellow physicians not to cut out stones but to leave it to the specialist. Nearer to our time, Samuel Pepys describes his own operation for the 'cutting of stone' on 26 March 1658. He notes in his diary that he spent twenty-four shillings 'for a case to keep my stone that I was cut of'.

Nephritis or Bright's Disease This was first described by Dr Richard Bright of London in 1827. The single disease which he diagnosed has now been subdivided into a number of conditions which may, in a broader way, be called nephritis – an inflammation of the kidney not resulting from infection in the kidney.

GLOSSARY

Calculus	a stone e.g. renal calculus – stone in the kidney
Catheter	a hollow tube which is placed into a cavity through a narrow canal to discharge fluid from the cavity, e.g. draining urine from the bladder for relief of urinary retention
Dysmenorrhea	painful menstruation
Ectopic pregnancy	development of the embryo in the fallopian tube instead of the uterus
Enuresis	involuntary discharge of urine
Foetus	the unborn child dating from the end of the third month until birth
Intra-uterine	within the uterus; relating to conditions which occurred before birth
Menopause	also called *climacteric*; the physiological cessation of menstruation
Micturition	the act of passing urine
Parturition	the act of giving birth

10 The Endocrine System

The endocrine system consists of a series of glands that secrete *hormones*. Although these glands are separate, they are functionally closely related and the health of the body is dependent upon the correctly balanced output from them.

Hormones are chemicals which cause certain changes in particular parts of the body. Their effects are slower and more general than nerve action. They can control long-term changes, such as rate of growth, rate of activity and sexual maturity.

The *endocrine*, or *ductless*, *glands* secrete their hormones directly into the blood steam. The hormones are circulated all over the body and reach their target organ via the blood stream. When hormones pass through the liver, they are converted into relatively inactive compounds which are excreted by the kidneys. Tests on such hormonal end products in urine can be used to detect pregnancy.

The endocrine glands

Endocrine glands are found throughout the body and include:

- the *pituitary gland*
- the *thyroid gland*
- the *parathyroid glands*
- the *thymus gland*
- the *hypothalamus*
- the *pineal gland*
- the *suprarenal*, or *adrenal*, glands
- the *sex glands*, *gonads*, in the ovaries and testes
- the *islets of Langerhans* in the pancreas.

The pituitary gland (Hypophysis)

This gland has been described as the leader of the endocrine orchestra. It consists of two lobes, *anterior* and *posterior*. The anterior lobe secretes many hormones, including the growth-promoting *somatotropic* hormone which controls the bones and muscles and in this way determines the

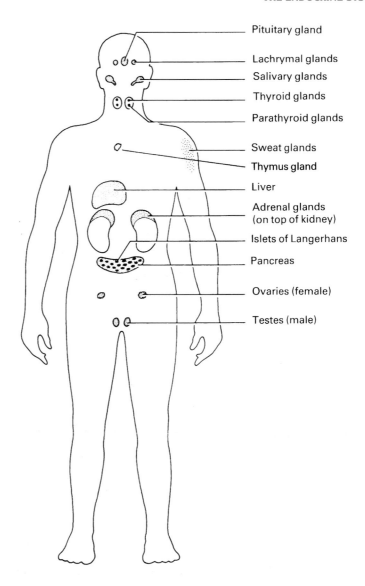

Pituitary gland

Lachrymal glands

Salivary glands

Thyroid glands

Parathyroid glands

Sweat glands

Thymus gland

Liver

Adrenal glands
(on top of kidney)

Islets of Langerhans

Pancreas

Ovaries (female)

Testes (male)

THE ENDOCRINE GLANDS
OF THE BODY

overall size of the individual. Over-secretion of the hormone in children produces gigantism and under-secretion produces dwarfism. The anterior lobe also produces *gonadotropic* hormones for both male and female gonad activity. *Thyrotropic* hormones regulate the thyroid and *adrenocorticotropic* hormones regulate the adrenal cortex. It also produces *metabolic* hormones.

The posterior lobe produces two hormones – *oxytocin* and *vasopressin*. Oxytocin causes the uterine muscles to contract during birth; it also causes the ducts of the mammary glands to contract and, in this way, helps to express the milk which the gland has secreted into the ducts. Vasopressin is an antidiuretic hormone which has a direct effect on the tubules of the kidneys and increases the amount of fluid they absorb so that less urine is excreted. It also contracts blood vessels in the heart and lungs and so raises the blood pressure. It is not certain whether these two hormones are actually manufactured in the posterior lobe or whether they are produced in the hypothalamus and passed down the

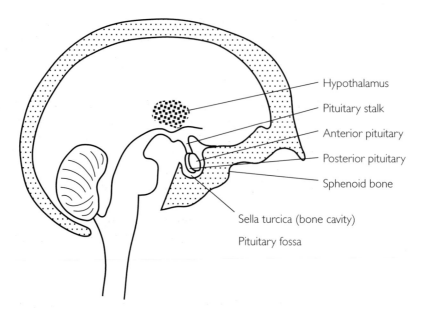

Hypothalamus

Pituitary stalk

Anterior pituitary

Posterior pituitary

Sphenoid bone

Sella turcica (bone cavity)

Pituitary fossa

THE POSITION OF THE PITUITARY GLAND

stalk of the pituitary gland to be stored in the posterior lobe and liberated from there into the circulation.

The thyroid

The right and left lobes of this gland lie on either side of the *trachea* united by the *isthmus*. The average size of each lobe is 4 cm long and 2 cm across but these sizes may vary considerably. The secretion of this gland is *thyroxine* and *tri-iodothyronine*. Thyroxine controls the general metabolism. Both hormones contain iodine but thyronine is more active than thyroxin. Under-secretion of this hormone in children produces cretinism; the children show stunted growth (dwarfism) and fail to develop mentally. Under-secretion in adults results in a low metabolic rate. Over-secretion in adults gives rise to exophthalmic goitre and the metabolic rate is higher than usual. Such persons may eat well but burn up so much fuel that they remain thin. This is usually accompanied by a rapid pulse rate. This gland, therefore, has a profound influence on both mental and physical activity.

The parathyroid glands

There are four of these glands, two on either side lying behind the thyroid. Their secretion is *parathormone*. Its function is to raise the blood calcium as well as maintain the balance of calcium and phosphorus in both the blood and bone structures. Under-secretion gives rise to a condition known as *tetany* in which the muscles go into spasm, and over-secretion causes calcium to be lost to the blood from the bones giving rise to softened bones, raised blood calcium and a marked depression of the nervous system.

The thymus gland

This gland lies in the lower part of the neck and attains a maximum length of about 6 cm. After puberty the thymus begins to atrophy so that in the adult only fibrous remnants are found. Its secretion is thought to act as a brake on the development of sex organs so that as the thymus atrophies, the sex organs develop. Recent research into the activity of this gland reveals that it plays an important part in the body's immune system by producing T lymphocytes – the T standing for thymus-derived.

The hypothalamus

This consists of a collection of nerve cells believed to form the control centre of the sympathetic and parasympathetic nervous systems. The hypothalamus releases hormones to the anterior lobe of the pituitary gland and neuro secretions to the posterior lobe. Via the pituitary, it is also involved in the metabolism of fat, carbohydrate and water, with sleep, body temperature and genital functions.

The pineal gland

This is still not fully understood. However, it is believed to have a regulating effect on the pituitary through the action of light via the optic nerve.

The suprarenal or adrenal glands

These are two in number, triangular in shape and yellow in colour. They lie one over each kidney. They are divided like the kidney into two parts – the *cortex* and the *medulla*. The cortex is the outer part of the gland and produces a number of hormones called *cortico-steroids*. Their function is to control sodium and potassium balance, stimulate the storage of glucose and affect or supplement the production of sex hormones. The medulla or inner layer produces *adrenalin*, a powerful vaso-constrictor. Adrenalin raises the blood pressure by constriction of smaller blood vessels and raises the blood sugar by increasing the output of sugar from the liver. The amount of adrenalin secreted is increased considerably by excitement, fear, or anger, which has caused the adrenals sometimes to be referred to as the glands of fright and fight.

The gonads or sex glands

These glands are naturally different in men and women because they serve different, though, in many respects, complementary functions. In the female the gonads are the ovaries, and in the male the testes. Female sex hormones are *oestrogen* and *progesterone*. The male sex hormone is *testosterone*, though each sex produces a small quantity of the opposite hormone. The female hormones are responsible for developing the rounded, feminine figure, breast growth, pubic and axillary hair and all the normal manifestations of femininity and repro-duction. The male hormone is responsible for voice changes, increased muscle mass, development of hair on the body and face and the usual development of manliness.

The pancreas

The endocrine part of the pancreas consists of clumps of cells called *islets of Langerhans* which secrete *insulin*. Insulin regulates the sugar level in the blood and the conversion of sugar into heat and energy. Too little insulin results in a disease known as *diabetes mellitus*. This disease is divided into two forms, one which occurs before the age of 25, and another form which begins in maturity.

It is a very common disease. It is known that some half million people in the UK suffer from it sufficiently badly to need treatment, but it has been estimated that there are many more people in whom the disease exists at a sub-treatment level.

Drs Rankin and Best succeeded in 1922 in keeping a diabetic dog alive in their Canadian laboratory by injection of insulin. More recently, with surgery, it has been possible to contain this disease although the supplement of insulin is really a support treatment rather than a cure.

Some notes on the endocrine system

The quantities involved in the secretion of the various glands are minute. For example, the adrenal glands, which affect all the organs of the body, produce in a complete year not more than 1 g of hormone.

Some hormone deficiencies appear to be endemic, that is they are particularly prevalent in certain parts of the world. The best example is probably to be found in the diseases which affect the thyroid through lack of iodine. For example, endemic cretinism is common to the upper valleys of the Alps and the Himalayas where endemic goitre is also present, whilst the latter condition is to be found also in the region of the Great Lakes and the Valley of Saint Lawrence. In all these areas, which are deficient in iodine or iodine-containing foods, the authorities now usually take precautionary measures such as the provision of iodised salts in order to stop the development of the disease.

GLOSSARY

Addison's Syndrome	a condition due to adrenal cortical tissue insufficiency, characterised by hypotension, wasting, vomiting and muscular weakness
Amenorrhoea	absence of menstruation
Cushing's Syndrome	condition due to oversecretion of adreno-cortical hormones, characterised by moon face, redistribution of body fat, hypertension, muscular weakness and occasionally mental derangement
Hyperthyroidism	thyrotoxicosis, toxic goitre and Graves' disease or exophthalmic goitre: the body's physical activities are subject to a speeding up, whilst the opposite condition, *hypothyroidism*, is evidenced by a slowing down of the body's activities
Lesion	an alteration of structure or of functional capacity due to injury or disease
Menopause (Climacteric)	cessation of menstruation; the period in female development when the reproductive function comes to an end, linked to a decline in the supply of hormone secretions by the ovaries. This is not a disease – it marks another stage in the female progression through life

Premenstrual Syndrome	symptoms of depression, irritability, bloating, swelling and restlessness that occur for about one week before the onset of menstruation
Steroid	the generic name given to various compounds of internal secretions including the sex hormones
Syndrome	a group of symptoms and signs which, when considered together, characterise a disease

11 Accessory Organs

This chapter describes those parts of the human anatomy which do not fit completely into any one system although they may form part of it. These are:

- **the skin**
- **the eyes**
- **the ears**
- **the breasts.**

The skin

The skin is the largest organ of the body and has a variety of functions:

- a protective envelope of the whole body
- a physical barrier to foreign materials and trauma
- a temperature regulator
- a sensory receptor
- an excretor of water, toxins and salts
- a synthesiser of vitamin D
- a membrane for the osmosis of some materials, such as drugs and essential oils
- a protective barrier to ultraviolet radiation.

To achieve these functions the skin is a complex organ. As an indication of this complexity, it has been estimated that 1 cm^2 of skin contains approximately:

- 3 million cells
- 13 oil glands
- 9 hairs
- 100 sweat glands
- 2.75 m of nerves
- 1 m of blood vessels
- thousands of sensory cells.

It is therefore easy to see how healthy skin is indicative of good mental and physical health.

The average human adult is covered by about 1.7 m^2 of skin, varying in thickness from thin over the eyelids to thick on the soles of the feet. It weighs about 3.2 kg and provides an excellent protection against germs, as very few can penetrate unbroken skin. Normal body processes produce heat and most of this is eliminated from the skin by radiation to the surrounding air or by evaporation of perspiration.

The structure of the skin Microscopically the skin is seen to divide into two zones:

- the *epidermis*
- the *dermis*.

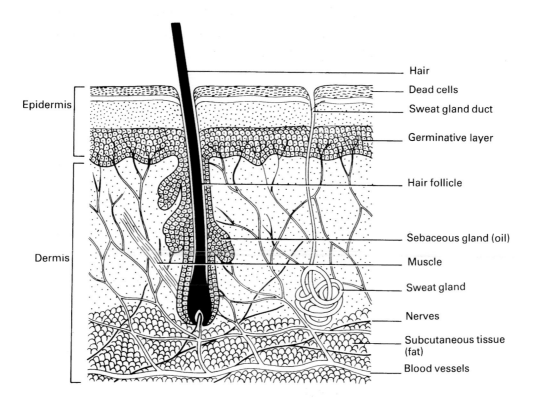

THE STRUCTURE OF THE SKIN

The epidermis

The epidermis (or outer skin) consists of five layers:

- stratum corneum
- stratum lucidum
- stratum granulosum
- stratum Malpighii
- stratum germinativum.

The outermost layer (the stratum corneum) is made up of dead flattened cells which are shed continuously as scales. Because so many millions of dead cells are washed or rubbed away every day, it is estimated that a new epidermis is created every 27 days – which is the birth to death span of these cells.

The dermis

The dermis (or true skin) consists of tough elastic connective tissue and is usually described as having two named layers:

- *the papillary layer*
- *the reticular layer.*

The dermis contains blood vessels, sweat glands, sebaceous glands, very small muscles (erector pili), hair follicles and tiny sensory nerves.

Subcutaneous fat lies beneath the dermis. It acts as a shock absorber, as an insulator to conserve body heat and is responsible for body contouring, which is more well-defined in the adult female body than the male. These fat cells may also be a source of energy in cases of food deprivation.

The sebaceous glands are small and found generally in all parts of the skin but are particularly numerous on the face, scalp and around the apertures of the nose, mouth and anus. They secrete *sebum*. A minor hormone imbalance can cause blocking of these glands giving rise to spots, blackheads and acne.

The odiferous or sweat glands are of two types:

- *apocrine glands*
- *eccrine glands.*

Apocrine sweat has more social than physiological significance. Apocrine glands are limited to a few regions of the body, primarily the axillary and genital areas. Inactive in infants, they develop in puberty and enlarge premenstrually. Freshly-produced sweat is sterile and inoffensive, but its decomposition by bacteria gives rise to perspiration odour.

Eccrine glands are responsible for the exudation of water, urea, salt and toxins. They are also involved in the vital heat regulating system that enables the body to keep a constant internal temperature of 36.8°C. They are especially numerous on the palms of the hands, soles of the feet and the armpits.

The sensory nerves of the skin register pressure, pain, itch, heat and cold and play an important part in temperature regulation. They relay information to the hypothalamus which houses two thermostats:

- One thermostat operates when it receives a 'cold' signal – it slows the flow of blood to the surface, restricts the activity of the sweat glands and shrinks the skin to form 'goose pimples'.
- The other operates upon receipt of a 'hot' signal – the blood circulation to the skin is stepped up and the sweat glands become more active.

The vascular system of the skin is based on a fine network of blood vessels (about 1 centimetre in a square metre of skin) and minute lymph spaces and channels.

Melanocytes cells in the skin produce the pigment *melanin*. This determines the colour of the skin, hair and eyes and is absent in albinos.

Melanin is a protective substance, screening out dangerous ultra-violet rays. When skin is exposed to the sun (real or artificially-produced), the pigment granules rise to the surface giving a protective tan. Freckles are concentrations of melanin.

Ergosterol is a chemical found in the skin which when activated by ultra-violet light changes into vitamin D, which is why vitamin D is sometimes called the sunshine vitamin.

The **erector pili** muscles are attached to hair follicles. They contract in response to cold and fear.

Nails are really appendages of the skin, being outgrowths from the epidermis.

The skin is highly elastic, as evidenced during pregnancy and obesity. It is mobile in most parts of the body, except where it is tightly bound down as on the scalp and ears.

The skin assumes different forms and shapes on the body. On the fingers and thumbs, it is ridged rather like a car tyre to enable grip, whilst over the knuckles of the back of the hand it is pleated to allow flexibility.

The skin is an excellent indicator of health and fitness – colour, pallor, dryness and flushing all being useful signs of what is happening in the body's physiology. Equally it responds to emotional and psychological stimulus as seen in blushing and dampness of the hands in nervousness or apprehension.

Whilst impervious to most substances, the skin will absorb certain drugs and essential oils. This function is being increasingly used in medicine, the active agent being placed under a patch on the abdomen or, in the case of anti-histamines (to prevent sea/car sickness), on the neck. The advantage is a more gradual absorption into the bloodstream, which is not chemically altered by contact with the hydrochloric acid of the stomach.

Some anthropologists and psychologists maintain that the skin is important in establishing relationships, e.g. the cuddling of a small baby by its mother transmits, through its nerve endings, a sense of affection and security.

Similarly, touch by massage can convey impulses of care and healing energies.

The eyes

Our sense of sight is the response of the brain to light stimuli which are received through the eye. The eyeball is a hollow, spherical structure, its walls consisting of three principal layers:

- the *sclera*, which is a tough fibrous, opaque coat, which is modified in front to form the clear, transparent *cornea*
- the *choroid*, or middle coat, which consists of an interlacement of blood vessels and pigment granules supported by loose connective

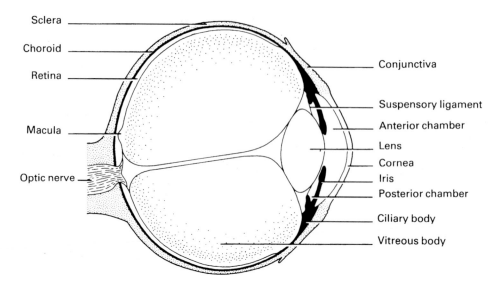

Sclera
Choroid
Retina
Macula
Optic nerve

Conjunctiva
Suspensory ligament
Anterior chamber
Lens
Cornea
Iris
Posterior chamber
Ciliary body
Vitreous body

THE EYEBALL

tissue. The *iris* is a pigmented, muscular curtain suspended behind the cornea. In the centre of the iris is an aperture known as the *pupil* through which light reaches the interior of the eye

- the *retina*, which forms the delicate inner layer of the eyeball. In this layer are found the *receptor* and *sensory* optic nerve endings sometimes referred to as *rods* and *cones*.

The eyeball has a number of appendages; the various muscles which directionally rotate it and the *lachrymal*, or *tear*, *glands* which moisten and clean the outer surface of the eye. Excess secretion of the lachrymal glands overflows onto the cheeks as tears. From the inner corners of the eyes the tears drain into a channel which opens into the nose, which is why weeping is sometimes accompanied by sniffing.

The pupil controls the light image by contracting in bright light and dilating in dim light. These light images strike the retina as an upside down image which is then conveyed to the brain through the optic nerve. The brain then reinverts the impulse so that it becomes a right side up image.

The ears

The ear is made up of three parts:

- the *external ear*, which consists of the *auricle* attached to the side of the head and the *external auditory meatus* leading from the auricle (or *pinna*) to the *tympanic membrane* or ear-drum. The function of the auricle is to collect sound waves and conduct them to the external auditory canal and tympanic membrane. The external auditory meatus or canal contains ceruminous glands which secrete cerumen or wax

- the *middle ear*, or *tympanic cavity*, which is a small air-filled cavity containing a chain of small bones – *auditory ossicles*. Sound waves are

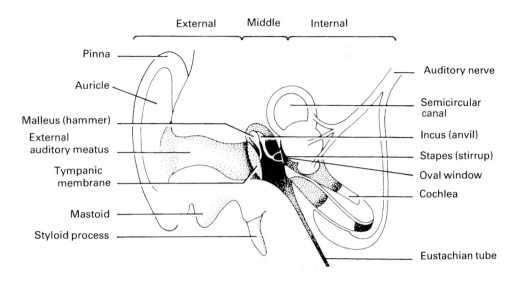

A SECTION THROUGH THE EAR

transmitted from the tympanic membrane (parchment-like) by the auditory bones (*malleus*, *incus* and *stapes*, popularly known as the hammer, anvil and stirrup) to the oval window (*fenestra ovalis*), a membrane connecting with the internal ear.

The E*ustachian* (*auditory*) *tube* links the ear with the nasopharynx to ensure that air pressure in the middle ear is the same as atmospheric pressure. The middle ear also communicates with the *mastoid antrum* and mastoid air cells in the mastoid process of the temporal bone

- the *internal ear*, or *labyrinth*, which consists of bony cavities (*osseous labyrinth*) enclosing a membranous structure (*membranous labyrinth*) which approximately follows the shape of the bony labyrinth. Between the bony walls and the membranous part of the labyrinth is a clear fluid – *perilymph*. This transmits the vibrations from the oval window to the *cochlea* (the essential organ of hearing) which connects to the brain via the auditory nerve. The *three semi-circular* canals (membranous canals or ducts) are situated in the bony labyrinth and control balance.

The breasts

The breasts (or *mammary glands*) are accessories to the female reproductive organs and secrete milk during the period of lactation. They develop during puberty, increase in size during pregnancy and atrophy in old age. The breast consists of mammary gland substance or *alveolar tissue* arranged in lobes and separated by connective and fatty tissues. Each lobule consists of a cluster of alveoli opening into lactiferous ducts which unite with other ducts to form large ducts which terminate in the excretory ducts. The ducts near the nipple expand to create reservoirs for the milk – *lactiferous sinuses*.

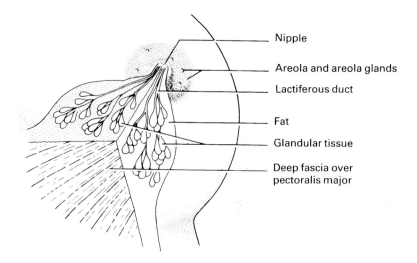

Nipple

Areola and areola glands

Lactiferous duct

Fat

Glandular tissue

Deep fascia over
pectoralis major

A SECTION THROUGH
THE BREAST

The breast contains a considerable quantity of fat, which lies in the tissue of the breast and also in between the lobes. It contains numerous lymphatic vessels which commence as tiny plexuses, unite to form larger vessels and eventually pass mainly to the lymph node in the axilla. The nipple is surrounded by a darker coloured area known as the mammary *areola*.

The breasts are greatly influenced by hormone activity. Hyper-secretion of the thyroid can lead to atrophy of the breasts, while hypo-secretion can cause greatly developed breasts. Both the ovarian hormones influence the condition and appearance of the breast, whilst the pituitary hormone, *prolactin*, starts lactation at the end of pregnancy.

Conditions and diseases of the accessory organs

Acne vulgaris
(Common acne)

This is one of the most common forms of skin disease. It is due to an over-secretion of the sebaceous glands and is invariably associated with the increase of sex hormones at puberty in both male and female. The primary lesion of acne is the *comedo*, or *blackhead*, which is darkened by air and not by dirt as sometimes thought.

Alopecia areata
(patchy baldness)

In this condition hair is lost from a small area, generally on the scalp but sometimes in the hirsute area of the face. There is no inflammation or any obvious skin disorder or systemic disease.

Cataract

The lens of the eye is situated directly behind the pupil and in health is clear. With age and in some diseases, such as diabetes, it loses its transparency and becomes more opaque, gradually shutting out vision – this condition is known as a cataract. It is not a growth but a biochemical change in the lens.

Conjunctivitis This is inflammation of the conjunctiva. In its acute contagious form it is known as 'Pink Eye'. It is caused by various forms of bacterial and viral infections. It includes swimming pool conjunctivitis and the type which is developed as a result of exposure to ultraviolet rays.

Eczema This is a term now used synonymously with dermatitis. It is not so much a disease as a complex symptom with many causes and clinical variations. There are a number of types or categories, their names, in many cases, indicating their suspected environmental or physiological cause. For example, lipstick dermatitis, perfume dermatitis, housewife's eczema (hand eczema) and industrial dermatitis.

Keloids These are rather like elevated scars and can occur after burns, cuts, scalds or surgical wounds anywhere on the skin.

Psoriasis Psoriasis is a common form of skin disease estimated to affect some 5 or 6 per cent of the population. It affects both sexes and is more commonly found in adults than children. It occurs in families sometimes and in about 25 per cent of cases it is hereditary. Psoriasis is characterised by the development of elevated reddish patches covered by a thick, dry, silvery scale.

Stye or Hordeolum A stye or hordeolum is usually caused by bacteria getting into the roots of one or more of the eyelashes, where local infection takes place. If, on the other hand, the infection gets into the sweat glands of the eyelid, a *cyst* or *chalazion* forms.

Tineacapitis

(Ringworm of the scalp) This superficial fungus infection of the scalp occurs in male or female before puberty and is characterised by partial loss of scalp hair and the breaking off of infected hairs. It is spread by direct contact with an infected person or through the use of a comb or headgear that has been worn by an infected person.

Verruca (Warts) There are many types of verruca, the best known being *verruca vulgaris*, or common wart, and *verrruca plantaris* which occurs on the soles of the feet. A verruca is a dry, elevated lesion which may appear singly or in large numbers. They are caused by viruses.

GLOSSARY

Acne Rosacea	unrelated to common acne; a chronic disease which affects the skin of the middle third of the face. It occurs most frequently in middle-aged women in whom it is associated with intestinal disturbances or pelvic disease
Antrum	a cavity or hollow space in a bone
Auditory vertigo	dizziness due to disease of the ears

Blister	a collection of fluid between the epidermis and the dermis
Colour blindness	a congenital inherited condition passed down by the female carriers to their sons
Hirsutism	a condition characterised by growth of hair in unusual places and in unusual amounts
Ocular vertigo	dizziness due to disease of the eyes
Tinea Pedis (Athlete's foot)	a fungal infection which is more common in men and more frequent in summer. In the acute form the blister type is the most common
Vertigo	giddiness; sensation of loss of equilibrium
Vesicle	a small sac containing fluid – a skin blister

GENERAL GLOSSARY OF ANATOMY AND PHYSIOLOGY

Acute	having rapid onset, a short course with pronounced symptoms
Anastomosis	the intercommunication of the vessels of any system with one another
Ankylosis	stiffness or fixation of a joint
Aplasia	absence of growth
Aponeurosis	the white, shiny membrane covering the muscles or connecting the muscles and tendons with the parts they move
Asthenia	the absence of strength in the muscles
Astigmatism	a defect in the focusing apparatus of the eyes
Bacillus	rod-shaped bacterium, e.g. tubercle b
Bacteria	single cell organisms without a nucleus
Benign	a tumour which is not malignant
Bilateral	on both sides
Biopsy	microscopic examination of tissue taken from a living subject
Calorie	a unit of heat that is the amount which raises the temperature of 1 kilogramme of water 1°C
Cardiologist	medically qualified person who specialises in the diagnosis and treatment of disorders of the heart and vascular system
Catalyst	a substance which greatly increases the rate of chemical reaction
Chronic	of long duration – opposite to acute
Coccus	spherical bacterium, e.g. streptococcus
Condyle	rounded projection at the end of a bone, forming part of a joint with another bone
Costal	relating to the ribs
Digit	finger or toe
Displasia	disordered growth
Dorsum	any part corresponding to the back, e.g. dorsum of the tongue

Dyspnoea	difficulty of breathing
Enzyme	a catalytic substance having a specific action in promoting a chemical change
Effusion	an abnormal outpouring of fluid (serum, pus or blood) into the tissues or cavities of the body
Electrocardiogram (ECG)	a graphic recording of the electric potential differences due to cardiac action taken from the body surfaces
Electroencephalogram (EEG)	a graphic recording of the minute changes in the electric potential associated with brain activity as detected by electrodes applied to the scalp surface
Filiform	slender – like a thread
Follicle	a small tubular or sac-like depression
Foramen	a hole
Fungiform	having a shape similar to that of a mushroom
Fungus	a plant-type infection, e.g. candida albicans
Fusiform	spindle-shaped, tapering both ways like a spindle
Gallstones	constituents of gall bladder which have crystallised
Glomerulus	a cluster of capillary vessels in the kidney
Hemiplegia	paralysis of half the body divided vertically
Hepatic	pertaining to the liver
Ingestion	the taking in of food
Keratin	proteins, the chief constituent of nails and hair
Lobe	a rounded part of projection of an organ
Lobule	a small lobe
Matrix	that which encloses anything
Melanin	pigment found in the cells of the skin

Micturition	the act of passing urine
Mitral valve	the heart valve between the atrium or auricle and ventricle
Myopia	short or near sight
Neoplasm	new growth
Neuroglia	connective tissue of the central nervous system
Neurologist	medically qualified person specialising in the diagnosis and treatment of disorders of the nervous system
Non-pathogenic bacterium	harmless to the body
Olfactory	pertaining to the sense of smell
Optic	relating to the sense of vision
Orthopaedic surgeon	a person who is medically qualified and specialises in that branch of surgery devoted to the prevention and correction of bone deformities
Osmosis	the diffusion of liquid substances through membranes
Osseous	bony or composed of bones
Paraplegia	paralysis of half the body divided horizontally
Pathogenic	disease producing
Pathogenic bacterium	disease-causing
Periphery	circumference; an external surface; the parts away from the centre
Peritoneum	the serous membrane lining the interior of the abdominal cavity
Physiatrist	a person who is specially trained in physical therapy especially for the promotion of health and fitness
Physiotherapist	a person who is specially trained in the science and art of physical medicine
Plexus	an intricate network of nerves, veins or lymphatic vessels
Psychiatrist	a person who is medically qualified and has specialised in mental or psychological conditions
Psychology	the science of the study of the structure and function of the mind; the behaviour of an organism in relation to its environment
Psychosomatic	a body/mind relationship

Pus	the thick white, yellow or greenish fluid found in abscesses, on ulcers or on inflamed and discharging surfaces, composed largely of dead white blood cells
Renal	pertaining to kidneys
Retina	the innermost and light-sensitive coat of the eyeball
Sarcoma	a malignant tumour composed of cells derived from non-epithelial tissue, mainly connective tissues
Somatic	relating to the body
Spirillum	spiral-shaped bacterium, includes vibrio and campilobactes
Squamous	scaly or shaped like a scale
Stenosis	contraction or narrowing of a channel or opening
Symphysis	the line of junction of two bones
Tactile	pertaining to touch or touch sensation
Tricuspid valve	valve of the heart guarding the passage from the right atrium or auricle to the ventricle
Tuberosity	a protuberance on a bone
Unilateral	on one side
Vasconstrictor	a nerve causing constriction of a blood vessel
Vasodilator	a nerve causing dilation of a blood vessel
Virus	minute particle only active when inside a host cell

The Study and Application of Therapy Treatments

In no way does this section pretend to be an exhaustive study of the subjects under review, but rather an attempt to spell out the main principles involved in such a way that you can relate the value of one treatment to another in a particular circumstance, or know how best to combine treatments in a way which will be the most satisfactory.

Most of the subjects under review have had many books written about them and in much greater detail than is possible in a textbook of this kind.

If you wish to research more deeply into any one particular subject there are many books from which to choose, but the following chapters will give you a good grounding in the use of some of the more popular treatments in physical therapy.

12 Massage

The art of massage is probably as old as man himself, because to hold or rub an injured part is an instinctive reaction to the pain involved. In days gone by, massage was largely practised by a priest/doctor, and many people believe that the laying on of hands, rather than being a religious ceremony, was a practical application by the priest for the relief of pain and the acceleration of health in the tissues. There are a number of incidents in the Christian Bible and other holy books which may be interpreted in this way.

A brief history of massage

It is generally believed that the word *massage* derives from the Arabic 'mass' or 'Mas'h' meaning to press softly. We know from ancient writings that the Chinese had a system of massage at least 5000 years ago – as did the Hindus, the Japanese and, just a little nearer our time, the ancient Egyptians.

Amongst very early writings, it is interesting to note that 3000 years before the Christian era, Chinese priests said in the Kong-Fu:

'Early morning effleurage with the palm of the hand, after a night's sleep when the blood is rested and the temper more relaxed, protects against cold, keeps the organs supple and prevents many minor ailments.'

Or again, about the same time, the Hindu priests were writing: 'massage reduces fat, strengthens the muscles and firms the skin'.

However, it is to the writers of the Greek dynasty that we are most indebted for early records of the way in which massage was used as an important part of the system of medicine. In the year 380 BC, Hippocrates wrote:

'A physician must be experienced in many things but assuredly also in rubbing – for things that have the same names have not always the same effect, for rubbing can bind a joint that is too loose and loosen a joint that is too tight; rubbing can bind and loosen; can make flesh or cause parts to waste; hard rubbing binds, soft rubbing loosens. Much rubbing causes parts to waste, moderate rubbing makes them grow.'

This medical use of massage appears to have been transferred to the Roman Empire because the famous physician, Galen, who lived during the second century AD in Rome, was an advocate of massage in the treatment of injuries and certain diseases. He wrote: 'Massage eliminates the waste products of nutrition and the poisons of fatigue'. However, with the decline of the Roman Empire, it would appear that massage became less associated with medicine and more with the pursuit of pleasure so that massage, rather than being something that was practised by the physicians and their trained assistants, was an art applied to the Romans by their slaves as a substitute for strenuous exercise and to help reduce the effects of excessive eating and drinking.

During the dark days of the Middle Ages the scientific use of massage largely disappeared, though a general understanding of human nature suggests that it must have been practised in some form or other during these times and it may be that the only weak link in the chain is the lack of documentary reference for most of that era. It reappears again in writings in the sixteenth century.

In the early nineteenth century a Swede, Henreich Ling (1776–1839), developed a scientific system of massage and exercise based on physiology. We are indebted to Ling for our modern concept of Swedish massage, though many years were to pass before it was generally accepted by the medical profession as a form of treatment, and it was not until 1899 that Sir William Bennett inaugurated a Massage Department at St George's Hospital, London.

Swedish massage

Swedish massage may be defined as *the manipulation of soft tissue for therapeutic purposes*. It is traditionally performed with talcum powder and this is applied to the hands of the therapist (not shaken on to the patient), as its aim is to enable the therapist's hands to slide over the patient. Putting talc on the patient results in the movements of massage forcing small particles into the pores thereby inhibiting some of the effects which should be achieved.

Massage has both a physiological and a psychological effect. The various movements massage exerts, either individually or in combination, affect the skin, muscle, blood vessels, lymphatics, nerves and some of the internal organs, depending on the position and pressure of the movements involved. In general, the *pressure movements* result in a speeding up of the body's physiology, whilst slow, gentle *effleurage* has a soothing effect, calming the nerves and enabling the patient to relax.

When effectively applied, this soothing massage quite often results in sending the patient to sleep.

In this book, no particular method of employing these movements is laid down because it is recognised that the movements are used in various combinations for different techniques. In fact most tutors have their own techniques and you should be wary of comparing the value of one technique with another except on a physiological basis. It is therefore of great importance that you should understand the physiological effects of the various movements so that you have a clear picture of what you are setting out to achieve, can intelligently interpret the movements which you are taught by your tutors and eventually be in a position to create your own treatment for any unusual condition which may present itself.

It may, therefore, be said that the two most important things to remember about massage are:

- the physiological effects of movements – either separately or combined
- when not to massage – the *contra-indications*.

It is important to know when and when not to massage, and this often differentiates the amateur therapist from the professional. An amateur with much practice is often able to achieve a reasonable standard of massage, but what he or she lacks is the knowledge of how, why and where to massage, and why not and where not to apply it.

Before describing the movements, there are several important points to remember if you wish to become a good masseur or masseuse as distinct from a merely accurate one.

- It is important to establish a sympathetic relationship with the patient because, as already mentioned, massage has a psychological as well as a physiological effect.

- Massage should not hurt the patient except in those therapeutic treatments where the cause is known. Pain or discomfort should always be regarded as a warning signal: either the pressure applied by you is too great for the sensitivity of the patient, or there is a more specific reason for the pain and this should be investigated.

- You should stand as close to the couch and the part of the patient being massaged as is reasonably possible. Standing an unnecessary distance away induces back strain and unnecessary fatigue.

- Most massage is achieved by using the muscles of the forearm and hand and not by employing the whole of your body, which again only adds to the fatigue factor.

- The patient should be provided with suitable covering – usually in the form of a towelling robe or towel. There are, of course, exceptions, but it is usually only necessary to uncover the part of the patient's body which is receiving treatment at a particular time and to cover it up again when that part of the body has been treated. See the section on towel draping in Chapter 29, page 256.

- It is essential to maintain a correct, professional attitude towards the patient. See Chapter 29, Professionalism, Ethics and Patient Support.

- All materials likely to be used during the massage, talc, tissues, etc., should be set out and be close at hand before treatment starts.

- The patient's comfort and preferences should be studied as far as is reasonably possible – for example: it is advisable, if possible, to avoid having lighting over the couch in such a way that the patient, in a supine position, stares directly into it.

● Never expect a patient to do for themselves something which you could easily do for them; if a limb has to be moved, assist with its movement and, in particular, help the patient on or off the couch.

Movements

Just as there are many techniques in massage so there are a variety of movements. But, in practice, they can be condensed into six basic movements:

- *effleurage*
- *pétrissage*
- *tapotement*

- *kneading*
- *hacking*
- *cupping.*

Effleurage

Effleurage is a movement which is mainly done with the flat of the hand, with the fingers close together and, as far as is practical, the tips of the fingers turning upwards so that they avoid protuberances such as the knee. Effleurage *precedes* all other movements because of its relaxing effect, enabling the patient to get used to the therapist's hands, whilst it also *succeeds* all other movements because it increases the blood and lymph flow in and out of the area as well as relaxing the patient.

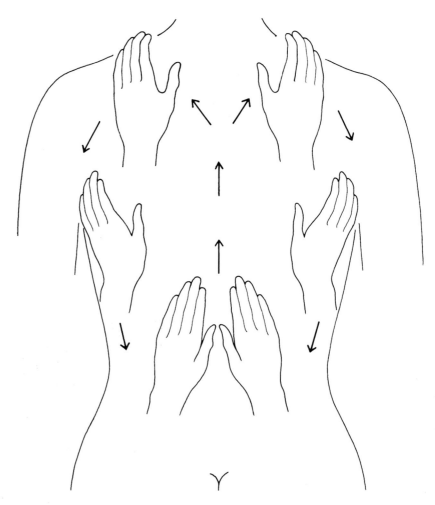

EFFLEURAGE

Effleurage movements are normally made towards the heart because – in addition to the effect of the effleurage on the skin and underlying nerves – it helps to speed up the venous and lymph flow. Effleurage should be reasonably slow and rhythmic, the same speed being employed in both the upward and downward movements with no break or interval between the two. The patient should experience one continuous movement but with a variation of pressure, which is on the upward stroke. This helps to induce in the patient a sense of euphoria or well-being. It is important in effleurage that the whole of the hand should be used and that it should conform to the normal contours of the body. When it is necessary to stimulate an area then quick effleurage is permissible. Stroking is a term which is sometimes applied to this movement.

Pétrissage Pétrissage is normally applied with the balls of the thumb and/or fingers and is applied to soft tissue that has bone immediately underneath it.

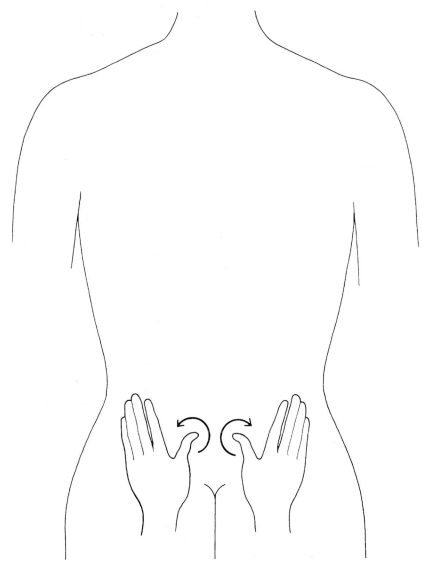

PETRISSAGE

In this way the balls of the digits are able to squeeze the soft tissue against the bone and so help to eliminate accumulated waste products. It is important in this movement to use the ball of the digit, not the tip, and not to slide over the skin but to securely trap it so that there may be a steady grinding type movement. *Friction* can also be covered by this heading.

Tapotement   These are fine, quick vibratory movements performed with the fingers of one or both hands. They are more often applied to the smaller muscles, for example those of the face, being used for their tonic effect. They are sometimes referred to as vibrations.

Kneading   Kneading is a very important movement because of its deep effect and because it can be applied to many parts of the body. It is normally used on soft tissue that has no bone immediately underneath it and its action is very similar to that of kneading bread. To knead an area satisfactorily the hands should be dry (with the application of sufficient talc to hands to achieve this) and the fingers should be kept straight – that is, in a tension position. The object is to pick the tissue up and away from the bone and to roll it back with a squeezing or pressure action. In this movement it is important not to press on the thumb but rather to use it as a guide. The effects of kneading are numerous. It particularly helps in the elimination of waste products from deep tissues especially muscular tissue. It assists in the breaking down of fat, improvement of body metabolism, muscle contractability and helps the interchange of tissue fluids. It is also decongestive in action. *Wringing, picking up* or *lifting up* can be included under this heading.

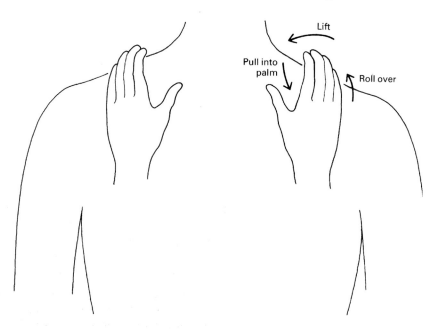

KNEADING

Hacking   Hacking is achieved with the edge of the hand, with the muscles of the hand in a slightly relaxed condition. If the fingers of the hand are too tense the result is a chopping action rather like a karate chop and this may be painful to the patient. Hacking is used primarily to improve the tone of the muscular tissue and is most generally used on the back, neck and shoulder area although it can be applied to other parts of the body. It has an effect on the larger muscles of the body similar to that of tapotement on small muscles.

Cupping Cupping is a quick movement achieved with the hands in a cupping position; that is, the finger joints are straight but the hand is bent at the point where the fingers articulate with the palm, and the thumb is brought in closely to create an almost airtight formation. When the hand is brought down on the body, the air which is trapped underneath is expelled, creating a vacuum which, when the hand is quickly taken away, sucks the blood towards the surface and creates a hyperaemia which is very good for the skin, the peripheral nerve endings and subcutaneous tissue. Like hacking, it is most often used on the back, neck and shoulder area but may be used on many other parts of the body. When properly applied it should sound like a horse trotting.

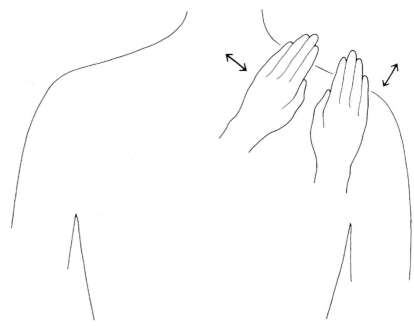

CUPPING

Exercises to improve
efficiency It will be clear that the above movements require a lot of practice before an expert touch is achieved. The following exercises will help to achieve this efficiency more quickly.

Exercise 1

Remove watch or bracelets from wrist and shake the hand quickly but as loosely as possible from the wrist until the whole hand appears like rubber. It is important that this shaking should only be from the wrist and not the whole arm. This should only be done for five to ten seconds at a time although it may be done several times a day. To do it for a longer period of time may only result in the stiffening up of joints instead of the suppleness which it is intended to achieve.

Exercise 2

'Throwing out the fingers': in this exercise the fingers are 'thrown out', that is they are extended and separated as far as possible in order to increase their strength. This should be done for five to ten seconds at a time but several times a day.

Exercise 3

This is an exercise for hacking. The elbows should be tucked closely in to the waist in order to prevent movement of the upper arm. The hacking may be done on a cushion or even on the front of your thigh. It should take the form of a quick, flicklike movement, the hands operating alternately. To start with, the speed will be slow but this may be gradually increased. If in the speeding up process the hands get out of phase with each other do not try to bring them back into phase but stop and start again. It should eventually be possible to continue this exercise at speed for at least one minute.

Exercise 4

This is an exercise for cupping and is treated in much the same way as the previous exercise – that is the elbows are kept close to the waist and the cupping is done on a cushion or on the front of your thigh. Other rules are the same as for Exercise 3.

Some additional notes on Swedish massage

Swedish or talc massage is suitable for most therapeutic treatments and for slimming treatments. This is because certain movements, particularly pétrissage and kneading, are achieved with much greater effect with talc as opposed to oil when the hands would be inclined to slip. Each movement is executed at least ten times and when done at the correct speed enables a whole talc body massage to be completed in about 50 minutes.

The following is a particular method of approach for a talc body massage. With the patient in a supine position, treatment is begun on the lower part of one leg proceeding to the upper part, then the arm on the same side. Walking around the head of the patient the arm on the opposite side is treated, then the leg, commencing with the lower leg. This brings you into a suitable position to treat the abdomen, waist and lower thorax. The patient then turns over to adopt a prone position and you, as you have remained in the same place, treat the leg, then the opposite buttock, then the arm and deltoid area, and walk round the head of the patient to treat the arm on the opposite side, then the leg, followed by the opposite buttock. This places you in a suitable position to undertake treatment of the back, neck and shoulders which concludes a full body massage.

Oil massage

It is sometimes mistakenly believed that the only difference between oil massage and talc massage is the medium used, but the difference is much more fundamental than this. In talc massage, your hands are talced so that they may slide easily over the body, whereas in oil massage the patient is oiled so that when pressure is applied the body tends to slide away from your hands. This means that in oil massage some movements have to be done in the reverse way to talc massage. For example in talc massage of the back, you apply effleurage standing parallel to the middle of the patient's body – that is, near the waist area and massaging with an upward pressure over the shoulders and back down again. To achieve this effect with oil, you need to stand at the head of the patient, applying pressure at the waist area and pulling towards the head.

Earlier in this section attention was drawn to the fact that certain movements like kneading are difficult to achieve with oil and that for this reason oil was not the immediate choice for slimming techniques. In addition, there is the fact of the absorption of the oil which many authorities believe provides more calories than it is conceivably possible to counteract by the slimming effect of the massage. Oil massage is, therefore, employed primarily for its relaxation benefits and is used in those conditions where the psychological effects are desired more than the physical ones.

The choice of oil is important. It should be a thin oil as thick oil tends to become sticky when subjected to the constant friction created by massage. It should be pleasantly but not highly perfumed, so that if used on a female patient, it will not clash with her own personal perfume and when used on a male it will not give the impression of being feminine. A number of good oils are marketed under the generic term *massage oils*. Bearing in mind that oil is primarily used for its psychological effect, the oil should be well presented and it is advisable to pour it into an aesthetically pleasant container rather than the plastic or other container in which it is purchased.

If you are specialising in oil massage, you should consider the advantages of *essential oils* treatment, provided you are qualified as an aromatherapist. Aromatic oils are chosen for their individual physio-logical effect and diluted in a suitable vehicle of vegetable origin such as avocado pear oil. A number of these oils are on the market and the manufacturers usually indicate the appropriate uses of the different types. Essential or aromatic oils tend to be expensive, but are extremely pleasant oils to use and the effect on the patient usually more than justifies the greater cost of the oil. In other words, these are normally used in costlier treatments – the increased cost being borne by the patient and not by you. For more information on the subject of essential oils (*aromatherapy*) the reader is referred to Chapter 26 of this book and to the author's book A *Textbook of Holistic Aromatherapy*.

After an oil massage it is very important that the patient should not leave feeling oily. This is normally achieved by wiping the oily areas over with paper tissues impregnated with cologne. When all surface oil has been removed a light dusting of talc is applied.

Holistic massage

The term *holistic* is generally interpreted as a treatment related to the whole person – body, mind and spirit. Holistic massage therefore has a variety of movements according to particular schools of thought, but in practice they normally incorporate the use of oil. Movements are slow and of light pressure and involve the whole of the body. Quite often music is used as a background aid.

Mechanical massage

Mechanical massagers fall into two principal types:

- *percussors*
- *gyrators*.

Percussors operate in a vertical plane; that is their movement is up and down and is approximately equivalent in physiological terms to tapotement or hacking. As the applicators are usually quite small, 2.5–4 cm in diameter, they naturally lend themselves to small areas of operation. Their use is limited to areas requiring tonic treatment and, when using hand-held percussors, to small areas. It must be pointed out that percussors come in a variety of forms, many of which are designed primarily for the home market. They include vibratory cushions, audio-sonic units, vibrating chairs and vibrating or massage belts.

Gyrators, on the other hand, operate in a horizontal plane and may be used to simulate the action of effleurage, pétrissage and kneading. Gyrators are sometimes referred to as *true mechanical massagers* because they approximate most of the actions undertaken by the human hand.

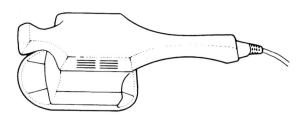

A HAND-HELD GYRATOR

Gyrators come in hand-held or pedestal form. The effect of both types on the human body is approximately the same – the choice being based on such questions as convenience and impressiveness. Gyrators are widely used in massage at clinic establishments and the reasons for this may be summarised as follows:

- They save time – complete body massage undertaken with a gyrator takes about 15 minutes against 50 minutes if the same areas were covered manually.
- Because less time is involved, massage becomes a more profitable treatment.
- Treatment is achieved with a smaller output of personal energy by the therapist.

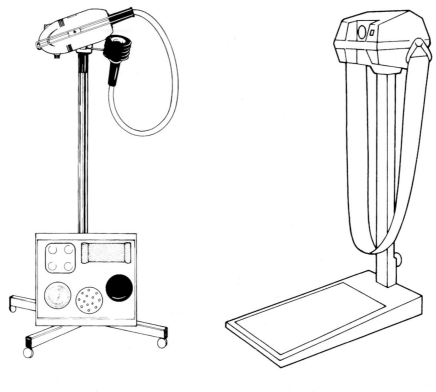

A PEDESTAL GYRATOR   A MASSAGE BELT

● The power and depth of penetration of the gyrator means that patients usually experience a deep sense of satisfaction arising from the feeling that their problems are being tackled vigorously.

However, it should be pointed out that, whilst complete body massage by means of a gyrator is a time-saving function, it lacks some of the aesthetic value achieved when the human hand is used. This makes combined treatments more popular.

Combined treatments

Combined treatments are those treatments which involve the use of gyrators on such parts of the body as the arms, legs and buttocks but use the hands on abdomen, waist, lower thorax, back, neck and shoulders. A treatment should take about 25 minutes. In a combined treatment the patient gets the best of both worlds – the power and depth of penetration of the instrument and the soothing, personal touch of your hand. Most of the movements in the normal Swedish hand massage may be simulated by the instrument so that mechanical massage is really Swedish massage achieved with mechanical aid. Together with the other advantages of combined treatments there is a saving of 50 per cent in the time involved.

One special word of warning – because of their power, gyrators should not be used over the abdomen or on the head, breast or genitals.

113

Most gyrators have a series of alternative heads or applicators. These are usually rubber or plastic in composition and therefore are in no way suitable for use with oil. Oil will not only cause the heads of applicators to perish but will cause a deterioration in the mechanism itself which is usually rubber bushed. Mechanical massagers may only be used with talc.

Another precaution to note is that hand-held models should not be run for more than about 15 minutes continuously – this is because they have powerful motors enclosed in a small area. Despite the fact that they have air circulating fans built into the mechanism, they tend to get warm in use. This is quite normal, but if they are allowed to get hot by continuous running for long periods of time, this will interfere with their efficiency and eventually cause a breakdown in insulation and necessitate repair and perhaps even motor replacement.

Contra-indications to massage

The following list does not claim to be comprehensive, but is rather a set of guidelines indicating the areas in which great care has to be exercised.

First and most important of the contra-indications is that therapists should not treat any medical condition except when referred to them by a medically qualified person.

Massage is contra-indicated:

- in areas of septic foci (because of the danger of spreading the infection)
- in contagious or infectious skin conditions
- over the abdomen during pregnancy (except with medical advice)
- over the abdomen during the first two or three days of menstruation
- in cardio-vascular conditions except with medical advice, e.g. thrombosis, phlebitis, angina pectoris, hypertension
- in areas of varicose veins
- over areas of unrecognised undulations (lumps and bumps)
- over recent scar tissue
- over areas of unexplained inflammation and pain (these should first be diagnosed by a suitably qualified person)
- any condition being treated by a medically qualified person unless he or she agrees.

Finally in any case of doubt do not hesitate to refer the case to a doctor for his or her advice.

GLOSSARY

Audio-sonic	percussor operating in the sound range, not to be confused with ultra-sonic.
Auto-infection	communication of disease through one part of the body to another
Contagious	the spread of disease by direct contact with the body of an infected person
Contra-indications	against, contrary or in opposition to its use
Infectious	spreading of disease through air or by other indirect means
Septic foci	principal area of sepsis, e.g. boils, carbuncles, any condition where pus is present
Traumatic	pertaining to or caused by wound or injury

13 Sauna, Steam and Other Hydrotherapy Treatments

There is nothing new in the use of thermal baths for the promotion of health. Public and personal hot air and steam baths were very popular in the days of the Roman Empire and the beginning of the use of sauna baths in the northern countries of Europe is lost in antiquity, whilst the hot water baths of the East, particularly Japan, were in existence many years ago. Thermal baths of the past were used for relaxation and socialising as well as for the treatment of disease and it is the purpose of this chapter to show how these age-old ideas are adapted to modern times.

Although achieved in different ways the principal effects of heat treatments are:

- *They are used to evaporate moisture from the body.* Most of this moisture is obtained from subcutaneous fat which consists of 65–70 per cent water. The amount of water lost from the body in this way can vary from 0.15 litres to as much as 1.5 litres in a single treatment. When combined with dietary control and/or supporting treatments this can result in a reduction in body weight.

- By *helping the body to perspire, they aid elimination of waste products and toxins through the skin.* The heat helps to activate the two to three million sweat glands which are in the skin. The liquid exudation from these glands, when subjected to analysis, is found to contain about 10 g of solids – 6 g of mineral salts, mainly sodium chloride (common salt), and 4 g of organic substances, mainly urea and urates. If the muscles have been actively working it also contains lactic acid which is the fatigue poison. It will be seen that this exudation is not unlike urine and its discharge through the skin is of considerable help to the kidneys. When sweat baths are used on persons ill from bacterially caused disease, the toxins thus created are rapidly eliminated through the skin – again helping overworked kidneys and reducing the risk of uraemia. The end result of this process of elimination is that the skin itself is thoroughly cleansed and left in a healthier, more elastic state.

116

- *They help the body to relax.* It has already been indicated in the anatomy section of this book that heat helps the body, and in particular the muscles, to relax and this is aided by the removal, through perspiration, of toxic products. There is also the psychological aspect of being warm, comfortable and looked after by someone else – in this case, the therapist. The combination of physical and psychological effects result in a deep sense of relaxation.

- *They prepare the body for subsequent treatment.* The success of many physical treatments can be conditioned by the state of the body to receive them. This is particularly noticeable in massage, vacuum suction and those treatments designed to aid relaxation. A warm body is a less tense body, the skin looser and the whole of the body easier to massage as well as giving more pleasure to the patient. Relaxed muscles are also more amenable to faradic treatment and the heat which softens subcutaneous fat makes vacuum suction easier and more efficient.

Contra-indications to heat treatment

These are not the limits of non-treatment, but a general guide to the type of conditions which should be avoided.

Firstly, no medical condition should be treated except on referral from a medically qualified person.

Heat treatment is contra-indicated by:

- cardio-vascular conditions – angina pectoris, valvular disease of the heart, history of thrombosis or arteriosclerosis
- abnormally high or low blood pressure
- congestive conditions of the lungs – such respiratory diseases as bronchitis or pulmonary tuberculosis
- skin diseases, except acne vulgaris
- persons who are under the influence of drugs or alcohol
- any person who is receiving medical treatment – except with a doctor's permission
- a heavy meal in the previous 2–3 hours
- severe exhaustion
- epilepsy
- persons who have not eaten at all for 5–6 hours, because of the giddiness which may result (This deficiency can easily be overcome by providing the stomach with some work to do with fruit juices or tea and biscuits.)
- diabetes – except with the doctor's permission
- the first 2–3 days of menstruation
- the later stages of pregnancy.

Heat treatment, equipment and method

Steam baths Steam baths were originally Roman or Turkish baths – sometimes they were intercommunicating rooms of varying temperatures so that it was possible to progress from cool to hot temperature or vice versa. Though a number of Turkish baths are still in operation, the term steam bath is now more usually applied to steam bath cabinets, that is individualised Turkish baths. These may be constructed of metal (usually aluminium), plasticised material or fibreglass. Although they vary in design the basic principles are the same, that is, a single seater cabinet with an aperture for the head and an electrically operated tank or evaporating tray for producing steam. Most cabinets have adjustable seats so that they are capable of accommodating anyone from a small child to a person 2 m (7 feet) tall. Most baths are fitted with rustless water tanks that contain sufficient water to give four to ten baths according to their duration. The heat can usually be controlled by two or three switches.

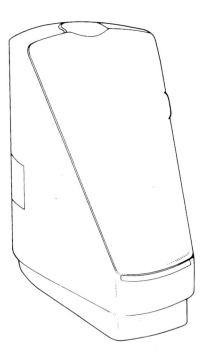

A STEAM BATH CABINET

Steam bath procedure

A typical treatment can follow this pattern:

1 The water level of the tank is checked to see that there is at least 5 cm of water above the elements.

2 The seat and its front are covered with towelling, the seat itself for hygiene and comfort purposes and the front to prevent steam getting on to the sensitive backs of the legs. A further hygienic

touch can be added by putting paper towels on top of the ordinary towels together with a paper towel on that part of the floor on which the feet will rest.

3 A folded towel is put over the aperture at the top of the bath to keep the heat in and the bath is switched on 10–15 minutes before required.

4 Having ascertained that there are no contra-indications the therapist takes the patient's towelling gown or towel that he or she is wrapped in, opens the door and helps the patient into the cabinet as quickly as is reasonably possible to avoid wastage of heat.

5 The towel which was blocking the aperture at the top is now used to wrap around the patient's neck, making sure that all the patient's hair is outside the bath and the timer is set for the required number of minutes. This can vary between 10–25 minutes – with an average of about 20 minutes, rather less for the first one or two treatments. However, these times must not be observed too dogmatically because if the patient feels uncomfortable he or he should be allowed to come out. Patients' tolerance to heat in a steam bath varies but 50–55°C may be taken as a reasonable average, that is for those baths fitted with thermometers, otherwise the therapist is dependent on the comfortable feeling that the patient is experiencing – having impressed on the patient that they should feel very comfortably warm – but not too hot. This is a point which should be watched very carefully because quite a lot of people feel that the hotter the bath the more effective it will be and this is not the case.

6 You may add to the sense of luxury of the treatment by occasionally wiping the forehead and/or face of the patient with tissue moistened in cologne or lavender water.

7 At the end of the scheduled time the patient is helped out of the bath and given a brisk rub down to remove the exudation which accumulates on the skin.

8 If the patient is undergoing other treatment he or she is helped on to the couch. If not, it is advisable for him or her to rest in a relaxing chair for at least 15 minutes before getting dressed.

9 If a shower is indicated, this should be warm not cold and taken at the end of the treatment or rest period.

Steam baths are not recommended more than every other day and twice a week is a reasonable average except in residential clinics where the patients are under closer supervision.

Sauna baths Sauna baths (pronounced sow-na) are usually available in two types: *panel sauna* and *log sauna*.

Panel sauna

Panel saunas are made of outer and inner panels of pine with an air space between. This air space is filled with an insulating material which serves the dual purpose of insulating the bath and thereby saving electricity, as well as preventing the heat escaping into the room and altering the room's normal temperature. This is particularly important when the sauna bath is part of the treatment room.

119

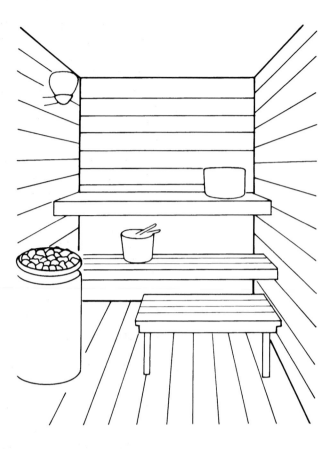

A FINNISH SAUNA

Log sauna

Log saunas are made of solid wood, slightly curved on either side to resemble logs and fitting into each other. They are particularly useful when a bath has to be specially made to fit into an area or alcove. This is not possible with panel saunas which are of pre-determined size. Heating is usually achieved electrically with stoves which have space on top for a quantity of special stones of a non-splintering type.

The smaller sauna baths are capable of being plugged into the normal household supply, but the larger ones require a special power cable similar to that used for electric cookers. A qualified electrician should be consulted before commitment to purchasing a sauna bath to ensure that the correct electricity supply is available.

The heaters are controlled by thermostat switches so that it is possible to pre-set to the required temperature. This control should be on the outside of the bath so that it may only be operated by you. Sauna baths usually have a free-hanging thermometer (which should be mounted as near to the top of the bath as possible), a water bucket and ladle.

Sauna bath procedure

A typical procedure for giving a sauna bath is as follows:

1   The sauna bath is switched on before it is likely to be required – about 30 minutes in the case of the smaller ones and up to an hour in the larger ones. Although the bath may switch itself off after say

15 minutes this does not mean that it has reached its maximum efficiency. This does not happen until the wood has absorbed sufficient heat to enable it to be re-radiated. Recommended temperatures are between 70–80°C – the higher figure being for the larger bath where there is a greater volume of air to circulate.

2 The seats may be covered with ordinary towelling or paper towelling and the pail filled with water.

3 Having ascertained that there are no contra-indications, the patient – who is normally just wrapped in a towel – is helped into the bath and advised to sit on the lower level until used to the heat, when he or she progresses to the higher level.

4 Treatment times are similar to those for steam baths, 10–25 minutes – with an average of 20. Some five minutes before the end of the treatment, the therapist adds water to the stones, sprinkling it by means of the ladle as rapidly as possible and quickly closing the door so that the vapour created in this way may be contained.

5 The patient is helped out of the bath at the end of the treatment period and subjected to the same routine as in steam baths.

As with steam baths it is very important to avoid overheating the patient because, here too, a lot of people believe that the greater the heat the more they will benefit and this is definitely contrary to the facts.

A recent review of sauna baths in Finland shows not more than 70°C to be the common temperature employed.

The practice of alternating periods in the bath with cold showers is to be discouraged. The heat of the bath dilates the capillary blood vessels allowing heat to escape through the skin and reducing the body's internal blood pressure. Subjecting the skin to a cold shower immediately afterwards causes the skin to shrink, closes the pores and pushes up the blood pressure, at the same time keeping in the increased heat. This is physiologically unsound as it subjects the heart to unnecessary strain. Repeating the process several times only adds further to the strain already imposed. In support of the cold shower or cold plunge pool, it is sometimes quoted that in Finland the participants in sauna are frequently rubbed with snow and that, as snow is not available in the slightly warmer climates, the cold shower or plunge is the next best thing. It should here be pointed out that the action of snow on the skin is very different from that of water, snow being used to treat people suffering from frostbite because of its friction qualities whereas cold water would exacerbate the condition. There is, however, very little danger attached to giving sauna baths providing that the correct procedure is adhered to.

Wax baths Wax baths are based on paraffin wax; there are several varieties. One example, 'parafango' is volcanic mud from the lakes of Northern Italy mixed into a paraffin wax base. Paraffin wax is a very suitable substance for heat treatment because of its capacity to hold heat and because the human body can tolerate a greater degree of heat in a paraffin wax bath than most other substances. Professional equipment is normally produced in two sizes:

- the small (or arm) wax bath which holds about 3.2 kg of wax
- the large (or foot) bath which holds 20–2 kg of wax.

A paraffin wax bath consists of an outer casing which accommodates the electric heaters and thermostatic control and an inner bath which contains the wax. The outer bath is partially filled with water thus providing more even heat for the wax as well as helping to maintain its heat at a constant temperature. If you only use this treatment occasionally, a very good alternative is to use a domestic double saucepan heated over a gas or electric ring providing care is taken to ensure the wax does not overheat. The temperature should be around 49°C.

Paraffin wax treatments are normally used for small areas, strains, sprains and especially rheumatic conditions. In residential clinics wax treatments are sometimes used more extensively, that is, for whole limbs and occasionally for whole body treatments.

Methods of application

There are four usual methods of application:

- The foot or hand is inserted into the bath and allowed to remain there for the period of treatment.
- The hand or foot is inserted in the bath and immediately taken out again; the air having a cooling effect on the wax creates a type of glove or sock. This is then wrapped up in towelling or blanketing to keep the heat in and this remains on for the period of the treatment.
- The wax is taken out by means of a ladle and spread on to a sheet of plastic to a thickness of about 6 mm. This is then applied much in the same way as a poultice to the parts to be treated and the whole wrapped up in towelling to keep the heat in.
- The wax is painted on by means of a brush and the part or, in some cases, the whole body is then wrapped up, first in a rubber or polythene sheet and then in a blanket.

Normal length of treatment is 15–20 minutes. When the treatment is concluded the wax peels off very easily without attaching itself to the hairy surface of the body and *hyperaemia* is revealed.

Foam and aerated baths Whilst these two types of bath are different, in effect the mechanism involved is the same. This consists of an air compressor and what is commonly called a 'duck-board'. At one time duckboards were made from a special type of porous wood but now they are invariably made of plastic perforated with hundreds of small holes. The duckboard is placed along the bottom of an ordinary domestic type bath and the electrically operated air compressor forces warm air through the duckboard holes. From here on the two methods differ.

Foam baths

The duckboard is covered to a depth of about 10 cm with hot water into which is put a quantity of foam extract, usually about 28 g but this depends on concentration. The compressor is then started and

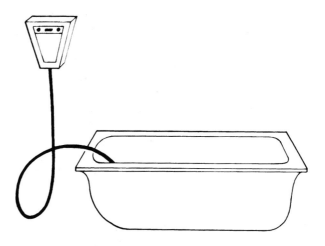

A FOAM/AERATED BATH UNIT

continues to run until the foam reaches almost the top of the bath, at which point the patient is helped into a lying position, as in a normal bath, so that only the head is outside the foam. By this time, of course, some of the water which was originally put into the bath has been used in creating the foam, so that the patient is only lying in about 5–7.5 cm of hot water. However, this is sufficient to generate heat in the patient's body and this heat tries to escape in the normal way through the skin. However, the hundreds and thousands of crisp bubbles act as very good insulation and prevent the heat from escaping so that it builds up on the surface of the body. This, in turn, induces more perspiration and the ultimate effect is very similar to that of a steam bath. The normal length of time is 15–20 minutes after which time the patient is taken out, given a warm shower to remove all the clinging foam particles and

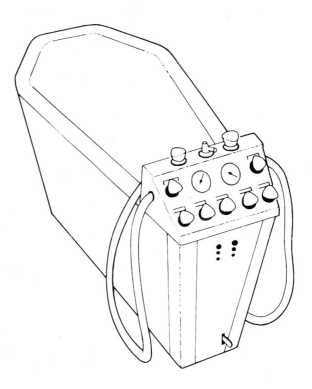

A HYDROMATIC BATH

then given a brisk rub down, following by treatment or 15 minutes or so of relaxation.

Aerated baths

Here the bath is filled with the normal amount of hot water required for a bath. Into this is put a quantity of seaweed extract, pine extract or other liquid extract of choice; the compressor is then switched on and the patient helped into the bath. By this time the whole of the bath is aerated, being superfused with oxygen, and the patient's body is bombarded by many thousands of little bubbles. The normal length of treatment is about 15 minutes, after which the patient is dried and proceeds to either further treatment or relaxation.

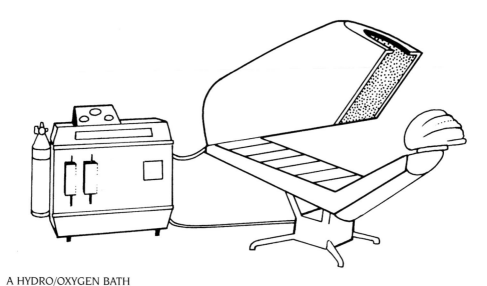

A HYDRO/OXYGEN BATH

Radiant heat baths Whilst at one time radiant heat baths were manufactured in cabinet form, they are now mainly constructed as tunnel baths. The bath, shaped rather like a tunnel, is made to fit over a standard massage couch and is normally fitted with 12 radiant heat bulbs. At one end of the bath are switches enabling the therapist to control the number of lamps switched on and therefore the amount of heat directing itself on to the patient. The tunnel bath is put over the part of the patient to be treated and the open ends covered in with blankets to maintain a good internal heat. In this way an excellent hyperaemia is produced but comparatively little sweating when compared with the wet heat or vapour bath. Treatment time averages 15–20 minutes but can be as long as half an hour.

Reference has already been made to the usual practice of relaxing after steam and sauna baths and then, if a shower is indicated, a warm one should be given at the end of the relaxation period. There are various reasons for this but the two principal ones are that the body continues to perspire for some time, in fact up to 30 minutes, after the conclusion of the steam or sauna bath and a shower would largely stop this process. Secondly, during steam and sauna baths the heart rate usually accelerates as do various other bodily activities, and a suitable period of either treatment or relaxation gives these a chance to return to their normal rate before the patient leaves the clinic and resumes normal activities.

14 Vacuum Suction Treatments

Vacuum suction in one of its various forms has played an important part in medical practice for several thousands of years. Second to massage, it must be one of the oldest treatments known to medicine.

A brief history

How far back in history the use of vacuum suction goes we do not know, but hieroglyphs found on the walls of King Tutankhamen's tomb when it was excavated suggest that the priest/doctors of Egypt used it and during the time of Hippocrates it appears to have been in extensive use.

An illustration of an early Greek cup shows that the vacuum was created by operating a plunger at the top of the cup. The Romans, on the other hand, obtained their vacuum in a rather different way. Inside the cup was a wick which was lit and the cup placed over the body. As the oxygen in the cup was used up, the wick went out; the hot air under the cup then cooled, creating a vacuum and sucked the tissue into the cup.

With the renaissance of medicine in the sixteenth century, vacuum suction became a popular form of treatment, the cups by now being manufactured of glass. Bell's cupping jars (nineteenth century) were still being used up to the middle of the twentieth century.

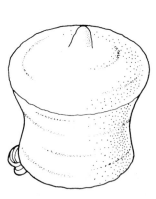

PRECIOUS METAL CUP – WICK TYPE
(ROMAN PERIOD)

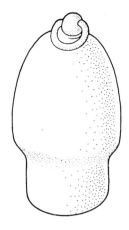

BRONZE CUP – PISTON TYPE
(PERIOD OF HIPPOCRATES)

A medical and surgical dictionary published in about 1865, under the term 'cupping', shows that the mode of procedure is first to exhaust the air from one of the glasses by inserting under it a flame from a spirit lamp and then immediately applying it to the body, when the skin is drawn into the exhausted receiver and the vessel is firmly fixed. After remaining on for a few minutes, the glass is removed by inserting the nail under the rim and permitting the air to enter, when it instantly drops off.

History records a number of variations in the method, especially when practised by country people who often used glass or earthenware vessels with wide mouths, such as jam jars, and heated them up either in hot water or by putting them in an oven. To have them at the right heat to create a good vacuum but not burn the patient obviously required a good deal of skill and experience. Today the vacuum is created by electrically-operated pumps and the vacuumatic or inverse pressure measured on a suitable gauge, so that whilst the method is very old the means of applying it is comparatively new and the number of purposes for which it is applied considerably increased.

Equipment

The equipment consists of an instrument, a series of cups of different sizes (usually 3 or 4 in number) and a plastic tube which connects the cups to the instrument.

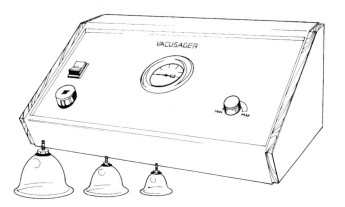

VACUUM SUCTION INSTRUMENT

Whilst the mode of construction varies with different manufacturers, the basic instrument normally consists of the vacuum pump, driven by an electric motor but more usually the pump and motor are an integral unit. The vacuum thus created is measured by a gauge which is normally calibrated in percentages. Scientifically vacuum is measured in inches of mercury so it is important to note that the measurement of these gauges on therapeutic instruments is not in inches of mercury but in percentages. Some instruments are not fitted with gauges but have preset percentage positions. The suction is then applied to patient via the plastic tube and the cup.

Care of equipment

Normally these instruments require very little attention except for the exterior parts. The cups need to be kept thoroughly clean and sterile;

this is achieved by either keeping them in a sterile cabinet or wiping with a cloth or tissue impregnated with a suitable disinfectant. The connecting tube provides a good lodging place for debris, powder, superfluous oil, etc., sucked off the skin of the patient and this tends to accumulate around the walls of the tube. If cleaned regularly, say once a week, the tube is kept looking clean. If, however, it is allowed to go for a long time before cleaning, the deposits tend to go green and look unpleasant and unhygienic.

Cleaning is effected by immersing the whole tube in a bowl of warm water to which detergent has been added. Allow to soak for about 15 minutes and then run clean water right through the tube from the tap. If the tube has been allowed to go too long without cleaning and the deposit has become encrusted on the tube walls, soak the whole of the tube in a stronger detergent solution for about 30 minutes, then thread a length of string through the tube, tie a knot in one end of the string and pull this slowly through the tube, repeating if necessary several times until the tube is quite clean. Rinse in the way already described. The plastic tube is flexible but not very elastic so, in time, the end of the tube which fits over the cup handle tends to get loose. When this happens the remedy is quite simple – with a pair of scissors you cut about 2 cm off the end of the tube and refit. In time this shortens the tube to the extent that a new piece of tube has to be purchased but it takes a considerable time for this point to be reached.

Most cups are composed of perspex or plexiglass and are, therefore, tough and resilient. However if they should be dropped onto a hard floor and crack or chip they should be immediately taken out of service. Cracked cups are liable to give faulty readings and chipped cups may damage the patient's skin. Some instruments have additional facilities known as static vacuum as distinct from the more usual gliding vacuum. This is for use when the cup is to be kept in one place; the operative or active vacuum (being the greater) sucks the tissue up into the cup but when this is released – as it is by a time mechanism – there is just sufficient vacuum left to hold the cup on to the tissue so that it does not have to be done by hand. In the experience of the writer this is a facility which is not widely used as it would appear that the results normally sought in the physical therapy field are more quickly achieved by the gliding method.

The uses of vacuum suction

First and foremost, vacuum suction increases the lymph and blood flow and, for this reason, the cup is normally moved towards the heart and directed to the nearest lymph node. In the process, that is the picking up of the tissue, including subcutaneous tissue, and moving towards the lymph node, there is a natural tendency to break down the subcutaneous fat and to accelerate its absorption into the lymph vessels, the contents of which are taken to the lymph node. The fat saturated lymph eventually arrives at the thoracic duct or the right lymphatic duct from whence it is passed into the blood stream where it may be used for heat or energy.

Vacuum suction is therefore a useful means of spot slimming but can, obviously, only be successful when combined with a calorie reduced diet otherwise the fat which has been released into the circulatory system becomes superfluous and is redeposited. Vacuum suction has another particular value in physical therapy – the reduction of trauma-produced oedema and accelerating the absorption of inter-muscular and subcutaneous infiltrates. It is emphasised that the oedema referred to is the kind caused by athletic and industrial injuries involving sprains, strains, contusions, bursitis and sinovitis and not the oedema that is of organic origin such as renal or cardiac disfunction.

The effects of vacuum suction may therefore be summarised as follows:

- increased blood and lymph flow
- production of hyperaemia
- stimulated metabolism
- improved absorption of intermuscular infiltrates.

This list indicates that vacuum suction may reasonably be used for conditions which come within the following categories:

- muscle toning, including post-traumatic and post-natal
- sluggish circulatory troubles (such as chilblains)
- reduction of oedema
- muscular and soft tissue that is overloaded with waste products (such as after prolonged athletic activity, certain forms of fibrositis, etc.)
- for accelerating reduction of subcutaneous fat.

Contra-indications to vacuum suction

Vacuum suction is contra-indicated:

- for the treatment of any medical condition until it has been diagnosed by a qualified medical person
- by any condition which is being treated by a doctor
- over or very near recent scar tissue
- over varicose veins
- on any person who has a history of thrombosis
- on an area which has suffered from phlebitis
- over or near parts affected by inflammation or septic foci
- over or near any infectious skin condition
- over the abdomen during the first 2–3 days of menstruation
- over the abdomen during pregnancy
- over the abdomen of anyone prone to hernia.

Notes on the contra-indications

Scars

A question which often arises is 'How old must a scar be before the area can be treated?' There can be no hard and fast rule about this, but the general guideline is that if the scar is a very small one, as is often seen in modern appendectomy, the area can be treated after about six months. However, if the scar is large, such as seen in hysterectomies and caesarian section, the area can be treated after about two years, unless the patient's doctor or surgeon advises it earlier.

Varicose veins

Whilst vacuum suction may not be applied over a vein, it may very usefully be applied above the vein – that is between the vein and the heart as the suction effect produced will help to empty the vein and so relieve the sluggish circulation which is normally associated with varicosity.

Method of treatment

1 Ensure the patient is lying in a position that is comfortable and the muscles relaxed as far as possible.

2 The area to be treated should be covered with a film of oil. There are several excellent oils on the market suitable for the purpose but, if for any reason these are not available, liquid paraffin may be used. Avoid, if possible, such oils as olive oil, sunflower oil, corn oil or castor oil because these tend to become sticky with the constant movement of the cup over the skin and this tends to pull the skin and be uncomfortable to the patient.

3 If the patient is wearing any underclothes make sure they are protected by paper tissues to prevent them from becoming soiled with the oil.

4 Select a cup of suitable size – this should be materially smaller than the part to be treated (as a guide, cup No. 3 for not too fat thighs; cup No. 4 for large ones).

5 Switch on the instrument and allow about 30 seconds for the motor to warm up if it is the first treatment of the day or the room is a bit cold.

6 Put a thumb completely over the hole in the centre of the cup thus stopping any air flow and with the other hand turn the power output control until the gauge measures the amount of vacuum required. (This action is not necessary when using a preset instrument.)

7 The cup is then put at the most distal part to be treated directly on top of the oil until the soft tissue elevates into the cup.

8 The tissue is then lifted and slowly moved until the cup is over the lymphatic node, care being taken to keep the cup in a level plane during the whole of the movement.

9 When reaching the lymph node the little finger of the hand holding the cup is pulled underneath the cup so as to break the vacuum

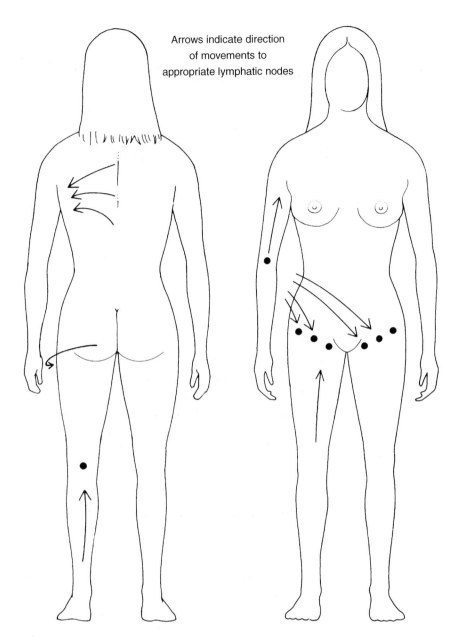

Arrows indicate direction
of movements to
appropriate lymphatic nodes

VACUUMATIC GLIDING
TREATMENTS (VACUSAGER)

and the cup returned to the distal area again. This movement is
repeated a minimum of six times.

10 The position is then altered by half the width of the cup, and six
more slow movements are made. This process is repeated until the
whole area has been covered.

It is important when breaking the vacuum over the lymphatic node
not to tilt the cup as this could result in broken capillaries. The
vacuum may only be broken by using the trailing finger method
already described or by inserting the tip of the finger of the other
hand under the cup. It is also important not to press on a cup
during treatment as this could be uncomfortable for the patient.

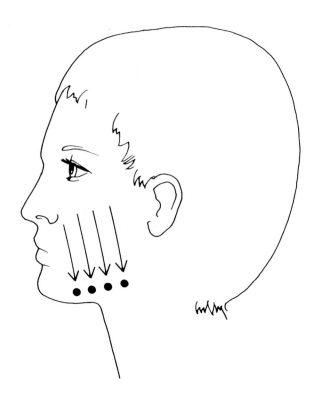

VACUUMATIC GLIDING
TREATMENTS (CONTINUED)

When learning this technique it might be useful to remember the following order:

- cup on
- lift
- move
- break.

11 At the end of the treatment all traces of oil should be removed with cologne or tonic lotion and then a sprinkling of powder.

In choosing the starting vacuum, attention must be paid to the age and condition of the patient. Experience will soon indicate the correct starting vacuum percentages but the following may prove a useful guide until the experience has been achieved:

- for young, healthy persons with elastic skin a starting vacuum of 8 per cent
- for middle aged persons or those of delicate disposition 6–7 per cent
- for old people with parchment type skin 5 per cent.

In all these cases the initial percentage should be reduced by 1 per cent when treating the sensitive areas of the body, that is the inner aspects of the thighs and arms, the face or the vicinity of the breasts. This means that where the starting vacuum is 8 per cent these sensitive areas of the patient should be only treated with 7 per cent. Providing the treatment is given more than once a week the vacuum may be increased each time by 1 per cent until a comfortable maximum has been reached which should not normally exceed 15 per cent.

When the patient has been under treatment for some time the number of strokes may be increased from 6 to a maximum of 10. Treatments should be given a minimum of twice a week – once a week not being considered satisfactory because it is not possible to build up the treatments. The ideal is treatment every other day particularly at the beginning of a course. Because vacuum suction is a build-up treatment, the patient should be warned not to expect visual results from the first four to five treatments, which indicates that the patient should be booked in for a course of not less than ten treatments in the first instance.

One final note – this is not appropriate treatment for patients who are grossly overweight, but rather for those who may have accumulated subcutaneous fat in one or two areas.

15 Electricity in Treatment

All therapists who use electrical instruments should have a basic understanding of electricity, the precautions necessary when using it, and how to locate and remedy simple faults.

Introduction to electricity in the clinic

An electric current is a flow of negatively charged particles, *electrons*; the unit of current is the *amp* or *ampere* (sometimes written as A). There are two types of electricity:

- *direct current* (DC), which flows in one direction only, and is supplied by batteries
- *alternating current* (AC), which repeatedly changes its direction and comes from a mains supply.

An electrical current will only flow between two points if there is a force or *voltage* to drive it. The unit of electrical force is the *volt* (abbreviated as V) named after Volta. The usual voltage for household electricity is 240 V although this varies in different countries and cities. It is wise to check the voltage required before purchasing electrical equipment. This information may be found at the electricity meter through which the supply passes from the local electricity supply company.

The *power* required for electrical appliances is measured in *watts* (W in short), named after the inventor of the steam engine. It is equal to the current in amps (A) multiplied by the voltage in volts (V). In other words:

Power (in W) = Voltage (in V) × Current (in A)

It is therefore simple to work out the power required to run an electrical appliance from the voltage and current. Equipment constructed for 240 V operation and labelled 10 amp will require 240 × 10 (V × A) W to run, i.e. 2400 W or 2.4 kW (kilowatts).

The current flowing through the appliance can be worked out from the power and voltage, and from this the type of fuse to be fitted to the equipment determined. A 1000 W or 1 kW single-bar electric fire run on the mains supply (240 V) will require 1000/240 A (W/V), i.e. just over 4 A to function. The plug top should therefore be fitted with a 5 A fuse.

Electrical energy is equal to the power of an appliance multiplied by the time for which the appliance is switched on and is measured in *kilowatt-*

134

hours (kWh). This means that a 1 kW electric fire will use 1 kWh of electricity when switched on for 1 hour. Electricity is charged for according to the number of kilowatthours used by the customer, and the electricity supply companies' name for the kilowatthour is a *unit*. If electricity costs 6 p per unit, it will cost 6 p to run a 1 kW fire for 1 hour.

A single-bar electric fire requiring 2.4 kW to run will use 2.4 kW per hour, i.e. 2.4 kWh, or 2.4 units. At 6 p per unit, this will cost 2.4×6 p = 14.4 p an hour to run. Light bulbs which require less power to run than electric fires will cost less to run per hour. A 100 W or 0.1 kW light bulb will use 0.1 kWh and therefore cost 0.6 p per hour to run.

In general, heat-producing equipment (sauna baths, steam baths, radiant heat lamps) is more expensive to run than electronic equipment (faradic units).

Wiring a plug   Household electricity has two *poles*, *live* and *neutral*. In the heating and power parts of the circuit there is a third wire known as an *earth* wire. These are usually colour coded, all new installations being coded in the following way:

- the brown wire is live
- the blue wire is neutral
- the yellow/green wire is earth.

In the old installations the live is red, neutral black and earth green. It is absolutely essential that clinic equipment used on a patient is always connected to an earthed plug, that is a three-pin plug. It is also important that the apparatus or plug should be suitable fused – that is the value of the fuse should not be much greater than the maximum current (amps) for the equipment.

All therapists should know how to wire up a plug. The illustration below of a 13 amp square pin plug should help. On most plug tops the screws are marked L, N and E which corresponds with the socket into which they are going to be placed so that the brown wire goes to L, the blue

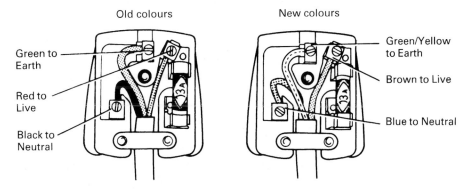

Old colours   New colours

Green to Earth
Red to Live
Black to Neutral

Green/Yellow to Earth
Brown to Live
Blue to Neutral

Remember: green/yellow wire to Earth terminal (marked E); blue wire to Neutral terminal (marked N); brown wire to Live terminal (marked L).

WIRING PLUGS

135

wire to N and the green/yellow to E. When the screws are tightened, make sure that the cord grip is screwed up firmly to stop the wire being tugged out and make sure that a cartridge fuse of the right value is inserted before you screw the cover plate back on to the plug top.

Fuses   It is important that you understand the purpose served by fuses.

In simple terms, a fuse is a piece of wire of known resistance. When the current passing through is too great the wire melts. So, for example, if the 1 kW fire (4 amps) to which we have referred earlier, is attached to a circuit which is fused for 3 amps, the fuse will blow (melt) because the current required to run the fire is greater than the fuse wire is able to stand. So, the function of fuses is to protect the instrument or equipment so that if anything goes wrong with the equipment, the increased current which it draws will blow the fuse. For example, if two wires get crossed, causing a short circuit, instead of burning out the equipment, as would be possible, the fuse is blown. It is important when a fuse blows to find out why it has blown because if this is due to a basic fault in the equipment or to wires touching in the lead or plug, renewing the fuse will be of no value since it will simply blow again. If, therefore, a fuse blows a second or third time in quick succession, it is always wise to have the circuit checked by a qualified electrician.

Fuse replacements are in two forms: wire and cartridge. Fused plug tops invariably use cartridge fuses and the fuses built into most modern equipment are in the form of cartridges. The mains fuses – that is those to be found usually near the meter – may be cartridge or wire. The more usual plug-type cartridges are 5 amp and 13 amp and it is always wise to keep a few of these handy in case of emergency. Wire is normally purchased on a card, suitably marked 5, 10 and 15 amp. It is also useful to keep a small screwdriver handy.

When mending a fuse on an instrument, make sure that the plug top is removed from its wall socket. It is not sufficient to just switch off. Before attempting to repair a mains fuse, always turn the mains switch to the 'off' position. If the fuseboard is marked in such a way that you can see which plug or set of plugs is served by a particular fuse then it is easy to locate the one that is faulty, but it is sometimes necessary to take out a number of fuse holders and inspect the wire to make sure that it is not broken or burnt before finding the correct one. When you have found it, remove the old wire and insert a new piece of wire of the correct amperage. Replace the fuse holder and turn on the mains.

Recent, modern electrical installations have *miniature circuit breakers* (m.c.b.) These are magnetically-operated when a fault occurs. The m.c.b. can be re-set by flicking a switch once the fault has been removed or rectified.

As a guide to the wattage a fuse withstands, and on the basis that the mains electricity is 240 V:

- a 2 amp fuse will take up to 480 watts
- a 5 amp fuse will take up to 1200 watts
- a 10 amp fuse will take up to 2400 watts
- a 13 amp fuse will take up to 3120 watts.

Safety precautions

- Equipment should not only be switched off at night but should also be unplugged.
- When fitting adaptors to plug sockets make sure that the socket is not overloaded.
- Never remove a plug from its socket by pulling on the cable.
- Do not expose electric cables to excessive heat. For example, do not run them too near a fire.
- Avoid trailing cables where they may easily be tripped over.

Battery-operated equipment

Batteries do not create electricity – they store it and so make it possible for apparatus to be operated independently of a mains supply.
There are two types of battery in common use:

- *throw-away batteries*, which are of no use once their electrical energy has been used up
- *rechargeable batteries*, which are more expensive initially, but which can be recharged from household current using a battery charger.

Most units with rechargable batteries are supplied with chargers at the time of purchase, and sometimes the charger is built into the apparatus. On no account should a rechargable battery be connected directly to household current without a charger as this will destroy the battery.

Some battery operated equipment is fitted with a battery indicator but where there is no such indicator on an instrument it is reasonable to assume that the batteries are running down when the power control knob has to be turned up higher to produce the same effect as previously. If for any reason it is intended not to use a battery unit for a considerable time, the batteries should be removed. Where there is a choice, batteries of the non-leak type should be used. These are sometimes marked HP batteries and are a little more expensive than standard batteries but longer lasting and their leakproof quality prevents damage to the apparatus.

Medical currents

The three types of current used in medicine are:

- *Faradic* – an induced current named after Faraday who discovered the laws of electromagnetic induction
- *Galvanic* – which is direct current named after Galvani who, using electric batteries, first obtained evidence of its effect on frogs
- *Sinusoidal* – or true alternating current of the type we have in normal household electricity, so named because its flow represents a sine curve.

The frequency of such alternations is important for the satisfactory running of some electrical equipment and a check should always be made that the equipment has been constructed suitably for the available current. The more usual frequencies for alternating current (AC) are 50 Hertz, common in the UK and Europe, and 60 Hertz common in America. At one time, sinusoidal current was used as a treatment in its own right but the new techniques developed in the manufacture of faradic and galvanic equipment have, to a large extent, caused sinusoidal treatments to be superseded except in certain special categories. This chapter will therefore deal with the two currents popularly in use – faradic and galvanic.

Faradism

This is used primarily as a *muscle exerciser* because of the readiness of the muscle fibres to accept this form of stimulation. It is at its most efficient when the pads are placed at the *point of origin* and the *point of insertion* of a muscle. This obviates unnecessary wastage of current in surrounding tissue though, because of the conductivity of tissue, it is possible to operate muscles from pads which are placed some distance away from them. This accounts for the variety of pad placement diagrams that are published. All of these work to a greater or lesser extent but those which are based on sound physiological principles will obviously act more efficiently and with a greater economy of current.

In general, the two pads or pairs of pads which complete the circuit should be placed at either end of the muscle or group of muscles which are to be activated or – alternatively – over the principal nerve feeding those muscles at one end and the point of attachment of the muscle at the other. For example, a pair of pads placed at either end of the thigh will cause faradic current to flow directly into the muscles, whereas pads put on either side of the thigh waste a lot of the current before it is picked up by the motor nerve activating the muscle or group of muscles.

When muscles directly cut across the path of other muscles there is bound to be an effect on the second group. For example if treating the abdominis rectus by putting a pair of pads just above the symphysis pubis and the distal end of the sternum, some of this energy is bound to flow into the abdominis transversalis which runs at right angles. Therefore if another pair of pads is put on the right and left sides of the waist it will require proportionately less current than if the position had been reversed. In other words, the first pair of pads to be supplied with faradic energy will require a greater amount of current because of leakage and the second pair a lesser amount of current.

Whilst the output controls of most instruments are calibrated, 0–9 are the more usual ones, it must be remembered that these calibrations only indicate the amount of current which is flowing into the tissue and are no guide to the result you might expect. This is because the amount of current required to move a muscle is conditioned by three factors:

- the size of the muscle
- the amount of tissue that it has to pass through before reaching the muscle. (It should be remembered that subcutaneous fat acts as an insulator rather than a conductor of electrical energy so that a fat person requires considerably more faradic current.)
- the state of the muscle.

Little used muscles, ones lacking in tone or subject to fatigue, require more electrical energy to move them. This may be summarised as size, depth of muscle and tone.

The pads necessary for conducting faradic energy to the muscles come in various forms:

- *Metal plates* These are usually cut out of pure tin (because of its conductivity factor) and are placed on top of several layers of surgical lint, previously soaked in normal saline solution (salt water). This method is now less used for general treatments because of time and cost.

- *Semi-conductor pads* These are constructed of rubber which, in the process of manufacture, is impregnated with graphite or a similar substance which converts what would otherwise be an insulating material into a semiconducting one. These have the advantage of being easy to apply, easily sterilised and long lasting.

- *Roller electrodes* These can be very useful especially on smaller muscles such as those of the face, hands and feet.

- *Handle* or *disc electrodes* which are normally only used when an individual muscle has to be tested or treated.

Faradic instruments Hand-surged faradic units – of which the Bristow Coil was the most common – have now been almost completely eclipsed by electronic instruments, where the surging is done automatically. There are so many faradic units available that it is only possible to give a short description of some of the principal types.

There are small, single or twin output units, usually battery-operated, particularly suitable for domiciliary treatments where only small areas have to be treated, for example part of one limb. Multi-output instruments are usually mains-operated though not always and come in

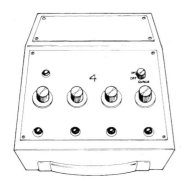

4 OUTPUT (8 PAD) BATTERY
OPERATED FARADIC UNIT

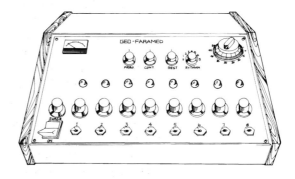

8 OUTPUT (16 PAD) FARADIC UNIT WITH ADDITIONAL
TREATMENT MODES

both transportable and clinic forms. These mains output units are especially suitable for physical therapists who undertake body toning treatments, and of these units the 6-output one is probably the type in most popular use. This has controls for six pairs of pads enabling the whole body to be treated, both legs, both arms, waist and abdomen.

There are individual differences in machines of different manufacture. Some have a fixed surge rate and function at around 50 surges a minute. Most of the medically-orientated instruments have a variable surge rate. All have individual power controls for each pair of pads – some have indicator lights which show when a particular circuit is live or in use. Some are completely transistorised in order to make them as small as possible and therefore easily portable. Some are mounted in large cases which may impress the patient. Whilst for the therapist seeking to specialise in this type of therapeutic activity, there are instruments with 8 outputs, individual power controls, variable surge rates, indicator lights coloured to match the patient's leads, variable pulse (useful in dealing with different disease conditions), a choice of current rhythms and variable rest times between the contractions.

There is therefore a wide choice of instruments from which to choose – instruments designed for the simplest to the most sophisticated of uses. It should, perhaps, be emphasised that in the multi-output units, not all the outputs have to be used at any one time so, for example, in muscle testing only a single output is needed.

Method of operation

1 Having decided which parts of the body are to be treated, the therapist selects the appropriate number of pads with their leads attached. The active surface of the pad (the part to be in contact with the patient) is well moistened with warm tap water.

2 The pads are then applied to the patient, being held in position with rubber or elasticated straps, and the leads then connected to the instrument, making sure that all the power controls are at zero.

3 The instrument is switched on and a suitable surge rate is chosen.

4 The power control of the first set of pads is then turned up until there is a visible contraction, then the second pair of pads is dealt with in the same way and so on until all the pads on the patient are producing visible contractions.

5 A timer is set for the length of time that the treatment is intended and when this time has expired, the instrument is turned off (so that all contractions stop simultaneously).

6 Each power unit is then turned back to zero and the pads taken off in the reverse order to that in which they were put on. This saves the wires becoming entangled.

7 The pads are then put in a steriliser or wiped clean with a disinfectant-impregnated tissue in readiness for the next treatment.

Surge rate

This is the rate at which the contractions occur and should be varied according to the condition or age of the person being treated. As a general guide, toning treatment for comparatively healthy, youngish persons can be in the 50–60 surges a minute range. In elderly people this might be reduced to 30–40 a minute. In post-trauma treatment, muscle atony or fatigue, it may be necessary to reduce the surge rate to 20 a minute or even less in some cases.

Time

This, too, is variable according to age and condition of the person treated. A healthy person could have, say, 15 minutes for the first treatment, 20 minutes for the second treatment, 25 minutes for the third and following treatments. Older people might start at 10 minutes and subsequent treatments be increased more gradually; in the case of injuries 5 minutes may be sufficient.

It should be remembered that Faradism produces passive exercise and is therefore capable of causing muscle fatigue, particularly in the elderly or those in a low state of health. It should therefore be administered with care and should be surge rate and time related.

For example, with the surge rate at 50 for 10 minutes the patient receives 500 passive exercises whereas with the surge rate set for 20 only 200 exercises would be involved in the same time. When receiving the first treatment, it is advisable to warn the patient that when the current is turned on the first sensation is a tingling not unlike 'pins and needles' but that as the current is increased this will give way to muscular contractions.

Pad placement for Faradic treatments

The diagrams below and on page 142 show the positions for pad placements. The broken circles indicate that the pads are on the reverse side of the body.

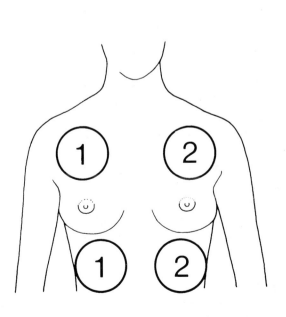

PECTORAL TREATMENT (BREAST UPLIFT)

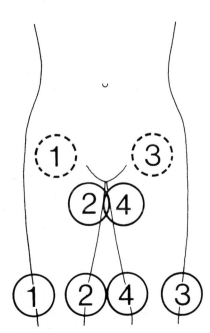

HIP AND THIGH TREATMENT

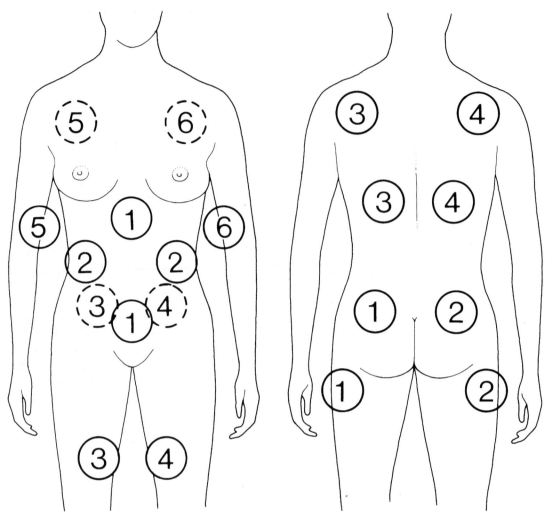

NORMAL FULL BODY TREATMENT

TREATMENT OF BACK, SHOULDERS AND GLUTEAL AREAS

Contra-indications to Faradic treatments

With the addition of muscle injury, the contra-indications are the same as those listed for vacuum suction treatment.

In summary
- Faradism is used to tone (or shorten) muscles by means of passive exercise. It is not weight-reducing in that it does nothing about fat, but by increasing the muscle tone it can make a part of the body look smaller.
- Surge rate may vary from 20 to 60 per minute.
- Length of time may vary from 5–25 minutes with an absolute maximum of 30 minutes, but at no time should this be continued to the point of causing fatigue to the patient.

- Current should never be turned up to a point where the contractions appear violent as this can do more harm than good. The contractions should be just easily visible.

Galvanic treatments

Galvanic treatments may be divided into two functions:

- *iontophoresis*, which is used with the current as a vehicle to transport substances through the skin into the body
- *deincrustation*, which has the effect of softening the skin, removing hardened sebum and clearing the skin of the accumulation of oil, traffic pollution and other debris.

The body is composed of cells, and cells, in turn, are composed of atoms. An atom is itself electrically neutral, but when it carries a charge it is called an *ion* – from the Greek meaning 'to wander'. Ions with a positive charge are called *cations* because they are attracted by the cathode or negative pole and ions with a negative charge are called *anions* since they migrate to the anode or positive pole. The unit of measurement used on galvanic instruments is usually the *milliamp* (one thousandth of an amp). The milliampmeter only registers when there is a resistance between the two poles. When the pads are in position the patient's body acts as the resistance, giving a reading on the meter, but when no 'body' is in the circuit there will be no reaction on the meter even if the output is turned up to its fullest extent.

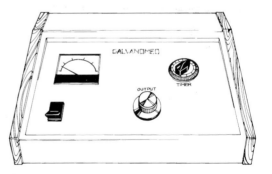

A GALVANIC UNIT

Iontophoresic treatment

This is body treatment where the galvanic current is used to carry certain substances, such as enzymes, into the body for physiological purposes, such as the reduction of fat, e.g. a suitable enzyme having an ingestive effect on the mucopoly saccharides. Because the material so introduced to the body flows to the anode or cathode, according to whether it is negatively or positively charged, it is important to ascertain this fact before commencing the treatment. Most substances supplied for this purpose are clearly marked.

Two metal plates are required, these are usually of soft tin and of a size suitable to the part to be treated, a size of 15 × 10 cm may be considered average – giving 150 cm² of electrode surface. In addition two pads of very absorbent material are required and these should be larger than the metal plates so that there is no possibility of the metal touching the skin. The absorbent material may be a number of thicknesses of surgical lint or the spongy type cloth of which there are several proprietary makes available. The one pad should be thoroughly soaked with the material to be introduced into the body and other pad soaked in ordinary water. A typical treatment would be as follows:

1 Massage the part to be treated so as to produce a hyperaemia.

2 Place the pad soaked in the material to be introduced under the *negative* plate, that is the one connected via the black lead to the black terminal on the instrument and the water-soaked pad under the *positive* electrode, that is the one connected via the red terminal.

3 Turn up the power control (which at this point should be at zero) very gradually until a prickly sensation is experienced by the patient, and then turn up even more slowly until the meter registers 2 mA. Treatment normally lasts 10–15 minutes when the power control is very gradually reduced to zero.

4 Remove the pads. It is a wise precaution to wash the area of skin that has been under the positive electric plate because in the ionisation process, acid and caustic alkalis are transported from the negative to the positive pole and tend to build up under the positive plate. Neither of the pads may be used again until they have been thoroughly washed.

The number of milliamps used for this treatment will vary according to the part treated and the sensitivity of the patient, but should be within the range 2–3 mA – this being the amount shown on the milliamp meter.

Deincrustation This is a method normally applied to the face. The material to be used is applied to the face in liquid or gel form. The electrodes, in this case, are usually rollers and these are attached to the negative terminal by means of black leads. The positive electrode is in the form of a rod or bar which is held by the patient to complete the circuit. A current of only a few milliamps is used and the electrodes must be kept constantly

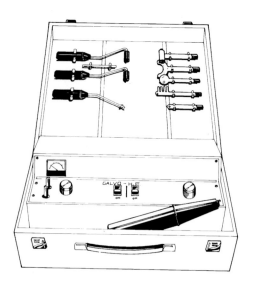

A COMBINED GALVANIC/HIGH
FREQUENCY UNIT

on the move – that is, in a rolling action over the face – but must never be allowed to touch each other.

As the aim of deincrustation is to soften and ease impurities out of the skin, the current must flow in the opposite direction to that of iontophoresis. This is achieved by putting the switch into the reverse mode. When using an instrument not fitted with a reversing switch, all that is necessary is to reverse the leads, i.e. to attach the red lead to the black terminal and vice versa.

During galvanic treatment, it is important that there should be no metal (jewellery or implants) within the area being treated. When the treated area is the face or neck, clients with metal teeth fillings may experience an unpleasant metallic taste.

For more information on beauty therapy treatments, you are referred to *Principles and Techniques for the Beauty Specialist* by Ann Gallant, also published by Stanley Thornes.

Contra-indications to galvanic treatment

Galvanic treatment is contra-indicated over:

- varicose veins
- pimples
- broken skin
- any area of septic foci.

If, during treatment, the patient experiences a hot sensation the current should immediately, but slowly, be returned to zero, the pads removed and the area under treatment inspected. To continue treatment under these circumstances can give rise to a galvanic burn.

16 Ultraviolet and Infrared Treatment

A physical therapist will come across several types of radiation:

- *visible light*
- *ultraviolet rays*
- *infrared rays*
- *sun-rays*
- *actinic rays*
- *radiant heat.*

These are all *electromagnetic rays*, or *waves*. They transfer energy from one point to another without any transfer of matter. The physical therapist is mainly concerned with visible light, ultraviolet rays, infrared rays, and waves in the short-wave range.

Introduction to electromagnetic rays

Electromagnetic rays are arranged in the *electromagnetic spectrum* (see the diagram opposite).

Electromagnetic rays have varying electric and magnetic fields which vibrate at different *wavelengths*, or *frequencies*. Frequency is measured in *Hertz*, or cycles per second. All electromagnetic waves travel at the same speed, so that as the wavelength increases, the frequency of vibration decreases.

Visible light

Visible light can be split into a band of colours – the light spectrum. This was first explained by Newton, who identified the band of colours red, orange, yellow, green, blue, indigo and violet as components of white light.

Visible light has a wavelength of about 1/2000th of a millimetre. The unit of measurement of wavelength in this part of the spectrum is the *Ångström unit* (Å). The Ångström unit is one hundred-millionth of a centimetre (10^{-8} cm, 10^{-10} cm). The wavelength of the visible light spectrum ranges from 3900 Å for violet light to 7800 Å for red light.

Ultraviolet rays

Ultraviolet rays cannot be seen by the naked eye and have a shorter wavelength than visible light. The ultraviolet band is approximately

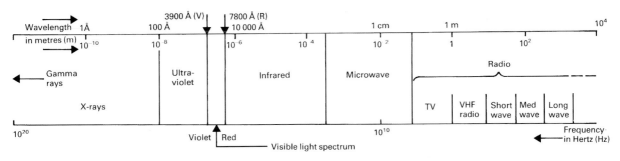

THE ELECTROMAGNETIC
SPECTRUM

250–4000 Å. Ultraviolet lamps used in physical therapy normally only operate between 2500–3300 Å.

Infrared rays Infrared rays have a longer wavelength than visible light. They produce heat but cannot be seen. They are referred to as *black heat*.

Sun-rays Ultraviolet rays have germicidal and cosmetic effects (see below), but as they are neither visible nor can be felt to be warm, some light from the visible spectrum and the infrared range is added to give bluish warm rays, known as sun-rays.

Actinic rays Actinic rays are rays occurring naturally in the sun which produce a chemical reaction, e.g. ultraviolet rays, blue and green light from the visible spectrum.

The therapeutic value of actinic rays was first discovered by a Danish physician, Niels Finsen, at the end of the nineteenth century. Known as *Finsen light*, it was a forerunner of the modern sun-ray lamp.

Radiant heat Invisible infrared rays can be made visible by the addition of some visible light to give radiant heat, or heat with light.

Ultraviolet treatment

The use and effects of ultraviolet treatment The physiological effects of ultraviolet rays vary, depending on wavelength and output. In general:

- Lamps radiating in the range 2500–2800 Å are *germicidal* in effect. They are used to create a bacteria-free environment, for example in ultraviolet sterilising cabinets or mounted over conveyor belts where it is necessary to have a high degree of sterility.
- Lamps radiating in the range 2800–3300 Å are *cosmetic* in effect. These are used in physical therapy, because of the effect on the skin.

Ultraviolet rays have two major effects on the skin:

- They activate *melanin*, a pigment which produces a healthy tanned appearance, which gives clients a sense of euphoria, or well-being.
- They activate *ergosterol* which produces vitamin D, which in turn acts as a calcium catalyst, important for the promotion of healthy bone structure. This is why vitamin D has been known as the anti-rickets vitamin.

Although ultraviolet rays may be used for a number of medical treatments, you are most likely to use them for these two effects.

Ultraviolet rays have one further use in medicine and that is as an aid to diagnosis. When a suitable tube is fitted with a Woods glass filter, it will cause certain skin conditions to fluoresce. This method is commonly used in the diagnosis of ringworm.

Equipment In the early days ultraviolet rays were produced by carbon arc lamps, but now most manufacturers employ the high-pressure mercury quartz tube or the longer fluorescent tube which is used extensively in sun-bed equipment.

Most high pressure mercury vapour tubes produce ultraviolet rays along the spectrum range and to cut out the lower end of this range, which is not normally used for physical therapy treatments, manufacturers employ two methods:

- In the bulb type generator the quartz tube is encased in a phosphate glass envelope which effectively acts as a filter, cutting out most of the range below 2800 Å, but allowing the cosmetic range to come through without alteration.
- The second method is to fit a sliding filter over the quartz tube. The manufacturers of such lamps claim that the value of a sliding filter is that, whilst the filter is over the quartz tube, you have radiation only in the cosmetic range whereas you can, if you wish, slide the filter off the tube so that you have the germicidal range which has certain treatment values.

Manufacturers often refer to the output of their UV products in terms of UVC, UVB and UVA:

- UVC is primarily the germicidal range and is eliminated in fluorescent tube units.
- UVB is in the melanin stimulation range.
- UVA, which is nearest to the visible light range, darkens the tan started by UVB.

Most sunbeds have a little UVB but are mainly UVA.

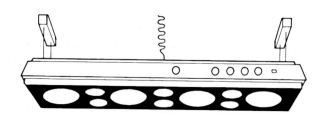

SOLARIUM CEILING FITTING
(ULTRAVIOLET RAYS AND
INFRARED RAYS)

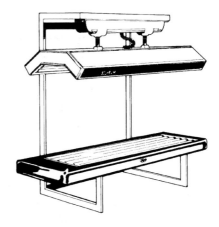

SOLARIUM (UVA SUN BED)

Method of treatment The aim of the first treatment is to produce a slight pinking of the skin (*first degree erythemadosis*).

The amount of radiation the patient receives depends on three factors:

- the *intensity of the light or radiation*, which depends on the power of the lamp, and as this is likely to vary, the manufacturer's instructions should always be consulted and strictly followed
- the *duration of exposure*, which is critical – if a patient is exposed to the light for 2 minutes, he or she will receive twice the radiation he would have received in 1 minute.
- the *distance of the lamp from the client* – the set distance must always be adhered to. If the distance is halved, the intensity of the light received by the patient increases four-fold (2^2); similarly, if the distance is reduced to one third of the original distance, the intensity increases nine-fold (3^2). This principle is known as the *inverse square law*.

The reaction of the skin to radiation differs according to the skin type of the patient and this must always be taken into consideration. Skin character is normally judged by the natural colour of the hair and is usually divided into three categories:

- average – all the so-called mousey-haired people fall into this category
- the natural blonde or natural redhead
- the natural brunette.

Dosage is normally based on the average type; the blondes and redheads requiring less exposure and the brunettes greater exposure.

If the history of the patient indicates unusual reaction to ultraviolet ray exposure then it is possible to do a patch test. An easy way of achieving this is to take a sheet of opaque paper, cut in the paper a line of holes about 4 cm in diameter and 1 cm apart, place this over the inner aspect of the forearm and mount the lamp at the standard distance. Expose the area to the ultraviolet rays for 1½ minutes then cover up the first hole. After a further ½ minute cover up the second hole and the third hole after an additional ½ minute. After a final

½ minute switch off the lamp. The arm should be inspected the following day to see which of the exposure areas most closely resembles a first degree erythema, which will then indicate the exposure time required for the whole body treatment.

All parts of the body being treated must be completely free of clothing and the skin free of oil or other skin covering. Before the lamp is switched on the patient must put on goggles of a special type provided for this purpose and such goggles must be worn throughout the treatment, whether the patient is directly facing the light output or not. It is *not* sufficient to close the eyes or to cover them with pads or material: both methods may allow sufficient ultraviolet rays to penetrate to cause conjunctivitis. The only acceptable precaution is the wearing of these special occlusive goggles the whole of the time the lamp is on. It is also advisable for the therapist to wear protective goggles because, although not directly under the light, he or she may be subjected to a certain amount of scatter radiation which will build up when there are a number of treatments during the course of the day.

The following is a typical treatment for ultraviolet lamps of the bulb type or those fitted with filters. The patient lies on the couch in a supine position and with protective goggles in place. The ultraviolet lamp should be exactly 60 cm from the patient, the distance measured between the lamp and the part of the patient nearest to it. In the female patient this is likely to be the breast area whereas in an obese man it would be the abdomen.

The patient of average skin type should be exposed for exactly 2½ minutes and then turned over into the prone position and exposed for a further 2½ minutes when the lamp is switched off and the goggles removed. If the patient is a natural blonde or redhead the treatment time should be reduced to 2 minutes whilst, for the natural brunette, it should be increased to 3 minutes either side.

Providing the treatment is given at least twice a week, each subsequent treatment may be increased by half a minute either side and treatment may be continued until a maximum of ten minutes either side is reached. When this point is reached treatment is either discontinued or, if the patient wants to keep up the achieved tan, radiation on the basis of once a week at the maximum dosage of ten minutes either side may be given. The patient should be told that there is not an immediate reaction to ultraviolet rays, but that such reaction usually occurs between one to eight hours after treatment when the slight pinking should become visible. This is sometimes accompanied by an itching sensation due to the drying action of ultraviolet rays but this can, to a large extent, be guarded against by the use of a suitable oil or moisturising cream after treatment.

Contra-indications to ultraviolet treatment

Ultraviolet treatment is contra-indicated by:

- all medical conditions except when under the direction of a medically qualified person
- congestive conditions of the lungs, for example bronchitis
- advanced cardio-vascular troubles, for example angina pectoris
- arteriosclerosis
- photosensitive skins, that is those skins which have an abnormal reaction when exposed to normal sunlight
- vitiligo, a condition in which patches of the skin are devoid of pigmentation
- skin diseases except under medical direction (skin cancer is itself associated with exposure to ultraviolet rays).

In patients with kidney or liver complaints, over-exposure can produce headaches, vomiting, nausea, faintness and insomnia.

Pigmentation of the skin to the extent that we refer to it as 'sun-tanned' is the body's natural protection against the admission of too great a quantity of ultra-violet rays, so that the more tanned a body is the fewer ultraviolet ryas are able to penetrate. It is worth noting however, that this pigmentation factor can be affected by drugs, some of which are widely used in medical treatment. If, therefore, the patient presents unusual reactions to ultraviolet treatment, their current medical condition should be checked in consultation with their doctor. Certain drugs and antibiotics sensitise the skin. *If in doubt, check with the client's doctor.*

Infrared treatment

It has already been mentioned that radiant heat is infrared rays plus some of the visible part of the spectrum. The physiological effects of black heat and radiant heat are almost identical, but there are certain practical advantages to be found in radiant heat which account for it being the more popular form of treatment. These advantages may be summarised as follows:

- Radiant heat generators normally reach their peak output 30 seconds after switching on, whereas infrared generators generally require up to 10 minutes to reach peak effect.
- Radiant heat lamps normally have a built-in reflector system which projects the waves from the lamp in a more or less parallel beam resulting in fairly evenly dispersed heating, whereas infrared generators depend on being mounted in a parabolic reflector and these tend to concentrate the rays in certain areas known as 'hot spots' which means that the heating is rather uneven.

151

- There is a certain psychological value to be obtained from the warm red glow which is given out by a radiant heat lamp as compared with the absence of light from infrared generators.

Infrared treatments are normally given for traumatic conditions such as sprains and strains and affections of joints and tendons, rheumatism and contusions. Even when its effect is not curative, the heat often has a soothing effect which is, in itself, often an aid to healing. Infrared rays have often therefore been described an *anti-inflammatory rays* and this is indicative of their main usage.

It is generally agreed that the physiological effects of infrared radiation fall into three categories:

- *hyperaemia producing*
- *relief of pain*
- *tissue relaxation.*

Hyperaemia In all local heating processes, hyperaemia is an essential factor including, as it does, the dilation of local tissue blood and lymph vessels and an increased flow of blood, which in turn brings in oxygen and nutriment. Congestion is relieved and the increased circulation promotes tissue repair.

Relief of pain This is fostered by the analgesic action of the rays on nerve terminals and by the relief of spasm and cramp.

Tissue relaxation The increased arterial flow due to the local application of heat causes the walls of the smaller arteries to relax and the vessels dilate, whilst the increased venous flow carries away a large quantity of waste products and toxins.

Method of treatment Unlike ultraviolet treatment, the duration involved in infrared treatment is not critical. It is generally agreed that 20–30 minutes is a reasonable period for treatment time, but this can be considerably exceeded without any deleterious effect. The correct distance from the lamp to the body is normally determined by the part under treatment being warm but not hot. If the treatment feels hot to the patient, the lamp should be moved further away. The patient should be warned of the dangers of tolerating greater heat in the mistaken belief that this will improve the value of the treatment. It may only result in a burn.

A typical radiant heat treatment would be as follows. Uncover the part to be treated, removing all bandages, plaster, etc., and make sure that the part is free of oil or embrocation. Switch the lamp on about 30 seconds before commencing treatment and position the bulb so that it is directly over the part to be treated and at such a distance that the part is comfortably warm but not hot. Treat for 25 minutes once or twice a day as required. Make sure that the treated part is not exposed to cold or draught after the treatment.

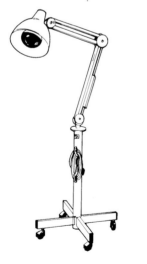

A SINGLE-HEADED TREATMENT LAMP (ULTRAVIOLET AND INFRARED RAYS)

Contra-indications to infrared treatment

- Particular care must be exercised in treating diabetic patients because of their reduced sensitivity to heat.
- Contact lenses must be removed before any treatment is given to the face, because they act rather like a magnifying glass in intensifying the heat.

17 · Exercise

All exercise is aimed at increasing the fitness of a part of the body, or the whole, and it achieves this by strengthening muscles, improving body metabolism and increasing the efficiency of the blood transport organs. Exercise may be undertaken without any external aids, or it is possible to employ various mechanical devices to assist the patient. Whichever method is used it is essential that these exercises should have rhythm and continuity – ten minutes exercise each day is very much better than sixty minutes exercise once a week.

It is not the purpose of this chapter to deal with self-activated exercise as there are many excellent books which deal with this subject.

Types of exercise

Exercise is performed in three ways:

- *passive exercise*
- *active exercise*
- *resistive exercise*

Passive exercise

We have already seen an example of passive exercise in the section on faradism – that is exercise which is mechanically induced and receives neither help nor resistance from the patient.

Another example is to be found in immediate post-trauma treatment when the therapist takes the limb and moves it such a way as to exercise the muscles involved but again without any help from the patient.

Active exercise

This is the second stage of post-trauma treatment and it is the point at which the patient is able to move the muscles himself or herself without any help from the therapist. Another example is to be found in a free cycling movement, that is, pedalling, but without any resistance.

Resistive exercise

This is the third stage in post-trauma treatment and this point is reached when the patient is able to accept a resistance against his or

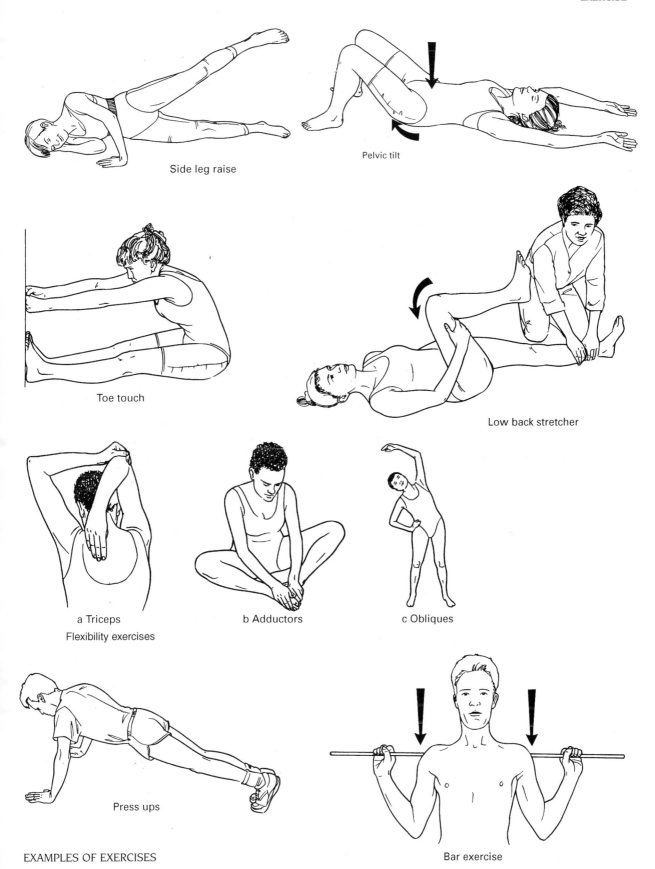

Side leg raise

Pelvic tilt

Toe touch

Low back stretcher

a Triceps

Flexibility exercises

b Adductors

c Obliques

Press ups

EXAMPLES OF EXERCISES

Bar exercise

her active exercise. An example of this is to be found when the therapist holds the limb in such a way as to allow movement but only against such resistance as he or she feels it necessary to exert and this is gradually increased as the injured part improves. Another example of this is found in a static bicycle which is fitted with a weighted flywheel or a resistance block so that the patient has to pedal against a load.

Mechanical exercisers

There are many aids to active exercise varying from a simple skipping rope to complex spring mechanisms, but a physical therapist is more likely to be interested in *ergometers*, that is, aids which have been designed for resistive exercise in such a way that the amount of resistance can be measured.

The two most popular forms of ergometer exercisers are:

- the ergometric bicycle, which is obviously most useful for the legs
- the ergo-rowing exerciser, which is especially useful for muscles involving the abdomen, back, shoulders and arms – but with useful leg exercises as well.

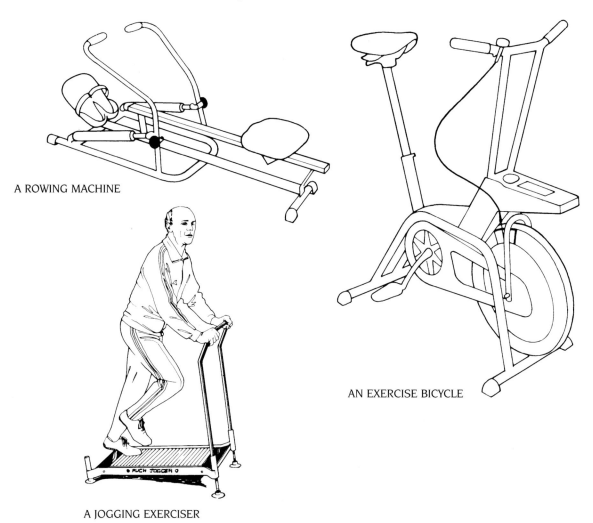

A ROWING MACHINE

AN EXERCISE BICYCLE

A JOGGING EXERCISER

The resistance is usually measured in kilogrammes or pounds and the more sophisticated bicycle ergometers are fitted with milometers and speedometers, whilst the rowing exerciser may be fitted with a movement counter. With an ergometer it is, therefore, possible to plan a complete programme of exercises, varying the speed, time and resistance. Whilst originally designed for muscle re-education and strengthening, ergometers are now increasingly used for keeping people healthy and, with this particularly in mind, the manufacturers usually also supply special programmes and advice on how their particular machine may be used in order to obtain maximum results.

18 Other Forms of Treatment

In addition to the treatments which have been described in some detail in the preceding chapters, there are a number of other electrical type treatments about which you should know enough to understand their function and how they differ from each other. These treatments are:

- *high-frequency*
- *diapulse*
- *short-wave*
- *microwave*
- *interferential*.

This chapter confines itself to an explanation of the *type of equipment* used for these treatments and the *physiological effects* which they achieve. Many excellent books are available which will provide you with more detailed information about these treatments.

High-frequency treatment

The term 'high-frequency', as applied to the apparatus usually known by this name, is in itself misleading. When they first came into use the currents *were* high-frequency, but they have now been superseded by much faster currents which really make them *medium-frequency* currents. The dividing line between low- and high-frequency currents is, in medicine, considered to be 100 000 cycles per second, because beyond this frequency no tetanus sets in.

The original work in this field was done by Nicolai Tesla who gave his name to the Tesla Coil. It was further explored and developed by the French physiologist, Jean d'Arsonval, who died in 1940 at the age of 89. The work to which we are referring was carried out mainly at the end of the nineteenth and beginning of the twentieth century.

Originally, the equipment involved was large and cumbersome and the patient sat inside a specially constructed spiral cage. Now the equipment is comparatively small and the current applied by means of

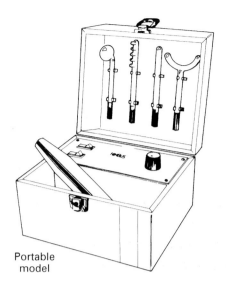

Portable
model

HIGH-FREQUENCY UNITS

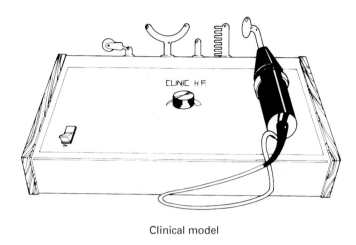

Clinical model

a hand-held applicator. Many claims were made for d'Arsonval's therapy but it is generally agreed that these may now be limited to a dermal effect. This falls into four categories:

- *effluvation*, which is contact treatment with one of the glass electrodes, used especially in those skin conditions where raising the skin temperature is of value

- *spark treatment*, which is when a glass electrode is held a very short distance away from the skin, sufficient for a spark gap to be created between the electrode and the patient. In this treatment the electrode is continuously moved over the area and in this way provides an alternative method of producing a gentle warmth in the skin under treatment

- *saturation*, so named because the patient becomes saturated with current. In this treatment the patient holds a metal bar or saturator after it has been inserted in the applicator holder and the therapist treats, with hands or fingers, a distant part of the body such as the face, the sensation being on the skin immediately under the therapist's fingers

- *fulguration*, which is a form of cauterising by using a special applicator. It is sometimes employed on skin conditions such as warts or verrucae.

It is important to note that whilst the patient is undergoing treatment he or she must not touch the machine in any way nor put his or her hand on any metallic objects such as metal struts of the treatment couch or chair. In both effluvation and spark treatment it is usual to apply a thin coating of oil to the skin before treatment.

Most of the glass electrodes emit a bluish violet light whilst in use, which has led to them being sometimes referred to as violet rays. They are not to be confused with ultraviolet rays because there is absolutely no connection.

159

Diathermy

Diathermic epilation is the method used for the removal of superfluous hair from the face or other parts of the body and the treatment is often known by its alternative name of *electrology*, because originally hair was removed by inserting a galvanic needle into the hair follicle. Whilst the galvanic method is still being used in obstinate cases, the more usual method is to use a short wave diathermy instrument with a frequency of about 27 000 000 cycles a second, that is, 27 megahertz. A cold light magnifier is useful when studying the hair follicle.

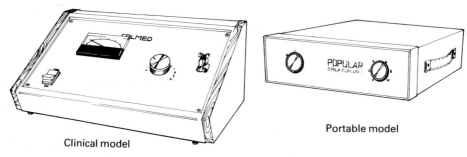

Clinical model

Portable model

DIATHERMIC EPILATION UNITS

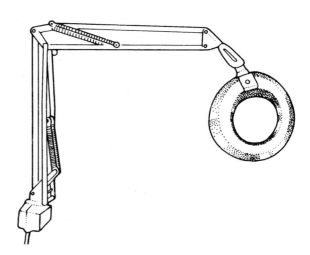

A COLD LIGHT MAGNIFIER

Short-wave treatment

When applied to the body, short waves provide heating in depth which makes them suitable for the treatment of joints and muscular tissue in particular. Application is normally in one of two forms:

● by rubber condenser pads which are placed on either side of the joint or part to be treated, with a thick separator placed directly between the pad and the patient's skin. These pliable electrodes may be moulded to fit the contours of the body and are held in place with rubber straps

160

- by means of air space electrodes. These are of rigid construction and again are normally placed on either side of the part to be treated leaving, in this instance, an air space between them and the patient's body.

Treatment time varies with the conditions to be treated but an average of 15 minutes may be considered normal. It is very important when using short-wave currents to make certain that no metallic objects appear within the field of treatment. This includes metallic jewellery or supports on the *outside* of the body and metal plates or pins *within* the body. The patient's leads, that is the cables which connect the instrument to the electrodes, must never be allowed to cross each other nor make contact with any metal object such as the instrument itself or the metal supports of a trolley.

Microwave treatment

Microwave is a mono-polar treatment, that is there is only one output head, and the electromagnetic oscillations are very much shorter than those of short waves, corresponding to a frequency of about 2450 megahertz. In short-wave treatment a good deal of the heat that is generated occurs in the subcutaneous fat tissue. This can be as much as ten times greater than that of the deep muscular tissue. With the very much shorter waves of microwave considerably less heat is created in subcutaneous fatty tissue and therefore proportionately more in the muscular tissue.

Treatment times are approximately the same as for short wave and similar physiological conditions are treated, but many therapists maintain that microwaves are easier to apply. As with short wave, metal must not appear within the field of treatment.

Interferential currents

Interferential current is really two frequencies slightly out of phase with each other. For example, if a frequency of 4000 megahertz has another frequency of 3900 megahertz superimposed on it, this gives a beat rhythm of 100 cycles, i.e. the difference between the two. The manufacturers of this type of equipment claim that very low frequency has a stimulating effect on tissue whilst, due to a decrease in skin resistance, higher intensities are possible. Beat frequencies of 0–100 cycles are the normal pattern of manufacture and reference books on this subject suggest the selection of different frequencies for a variety of soft tissue conditions.

Treatment using interferential currents also has an important role in pain management. For more information on this subject, consult *Interferential Therapy* by Brenda Savage, M.Sc., MSCP, published by Wolfe Publishing Ltd.

19 First Aid

This chapter is not intended to deal in detail with such an extensive subject, but rather to indicate guidelines for the treatment of some of the more common conditions met with in clinics and leisure centres. For further study, refer to the *First-aid Manual* (the authorised publication of the St John Ambulance, St Andrew's Association and the British Red Cross Society).

Fainting

This is a brief loss of consciousness created by a temporary reduction of blood flow to the brain. It has a variety of causes including exhaustion, lack of food, pain and emotional upset.

Treatment   Sit the patient down putting the head between knees and advise taking deep breaths. Loosen tight clothing particularly at the neck, chest and waist.

Bruising

Treatment   Raise the injured part to a position the patient finds comfortable and apply cold compresses.

Shock

This is sometimes accompanied by cold clammy skin and/or sweating.

Treatment   Be firm and positive with the patient and especially reassuring. Lay the patient down in a supine position with the head low on one side. Cover with a blanket, keep the patient warm and summon medical assistance.

Minor burns and scalds

Treatment   Place the injured part under slow-running cold water (or, if this is not available, immerse in a container of cold water) for ten minutes or such time as the pain persists. Remove rings, bracelets, etc. because of the risk of swelling and cover with a sterile (non-fluffy) dressing.

Bleeding

Treatment   Most haemorrhages can be controlled with a pressure pad or with the thumb and fingers. In the case of the former, a sterile pad should be used and bandaged firmly in place.

When the bleeding is from a varicose vein (usually a leg) lay the patient on his or her back, remove any constricting clothes and elevate the leg on a chair or suitable object. Arrange for the patient to be taken to hospital.

Heat exhaustion

The patient may have a headache and feel very tired and dizzy. The breathing may be fast and the pulse rapid. Cramp in the lower limbs is not uncommon.

Treatment   Lay the patient down in a cool place, provide sips of water and seek medical help.

Choking

Treatment   If the patient is conscious, coughing to dislodge the offending object may be all that is needed. If necessary this may be followed by a jolt to the back (back slapping).

If these fail then apply an abdominal thrust. This should be left until last because of the danger of injuring the internal organs. The abdominal thrust is achieved by putting one arm around the patient with the clenched fist thumb inwards between the navel and distal sternum. Grasp the fist with the other hand and pull towards you with a quick inward and upward thrust from the elbows. Repeat up to four times.

Fractures

Treatment In the case of a fracture of the clavicle or a shoulder dislocation, support the arm in a diagonal position with a sling, scarf or other suitable material.

With other fractures, immobilise and support in the position found. Do not attempt to straighten a limb where a fracture is suspected. Arrange for the patient to be taken to hospital.

Cardiac arrest

Treatment while awaiting medical assistance (This treatment also applies to other conditions where breathing has stopped.) Place the patient in a supine position with the head tilted back. Make sure that the airway is clear of loose dentures, etc. To stop the tongue obstructing the airway, the patient's neck needs to be extended. To do this, place one hand under the neck and the other on the forehead. The latter pushes the head back when the neck hand is lifted.

Leaving one hand under the neck, use the other one to pinch the nose. Place your lips over the patient's mouth making a complete seal and exhale into the patient at least four times in quick succession, then repeat if necessary.

It is advisable to practise this method so as to be efficient should the occasion arise. Contact one of the aforementioned organisations or other training agencies and join one of their classes on artificial ventilation.

Asthmatic attack

Treatment Put the patient in a sitting position with arms resting in front of them. Make sure that all clothing is loose and keep the patient warm. Gentle rubbing of the back often gives relief. Allow the patient to take his or her own medication if it is available.

The recovery position

An unconscious person must not be left lying on his or her back because of the risk of choking.

1 With the patient lying straight on the floor, place the arm nearest to you at right angles to the body, elbow bent and with the palm of the hand uppermost.

2   Bring the arm furthest from you across the chest and hold the palm of the hand outwards against the nearer cheek.

3   Grasp the leg above the knee and roll the patient towards you.

The patient should end up lying on his or her side, with the uppermost leg bent at the knee and the head supported by the uppermost arm (see the illustration below).

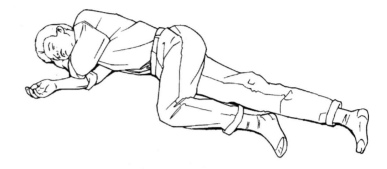

THE RECOVERY POSITION

> If you are in any doubt about the condition of the patient, or if the trauma is severe, seek medical assistance immediately.

Accident book

All accidents, however small, should be recorded in an accident book, giving as much detail as possible including:

- name and address of casualty
- nature of accident as observed at the time
- time of accident
- first-aid treatment given
- names and addresses of any witnesses.

First aid box

All establishments should have a professional-type first aid box on the premises. It should be easily accessible and kept fully stocked.

Specialised Aspects of Physical Therapy

Physical therapy has many specialised aspects and is increasingly recognised as playing an important part in the treatment of injuries and the promotion of fitness.

20 Sports Therapy

Athletics and leisure-type pursuits which involve vigorous exercise have been with us for a very long time. Recently they have taken on a new importance, partly because of the increased leisure which is available to most people and partly because of the way in which they have been linked to health in general and prevention of certain conditions of ill-health, in particular obesity and heart disease. As more people become involved in this type of activity, there is bound to be an increased number of injuries and it is estimated that up to 10 per cent of casualties treated in hospital fall into the category of sports-injuries. These injuries are not necessarily caused by sport but they do, however, fall into a particular category. It will be obvious that an ankle sprained by falling down stairs needs the same treatment as an ankle sprained on the football field.

This chapter aims to give guidance on the initial or first-aid treatment of sports-type injuries, it being generally agreed that correct treatment in the early stages can often prevent unnecessary complications and in this way considerably reduce the rehabilitation period.

Many injuries should, of course, have specialist treatment. Even with the slightest suspicion there should be no hesitation whatsoever in sending such patients to the nearest hospital, or, alternatively, to their own doctor who may be able to direct them to a specialist in sports medicine.

Sports medicine in itself is by no means a new speciality. At the time of the Greek empire much emphasis was placed on the fitness of young men and those who excelled at athletics were treated almost as young gods. Subsequently, special provision was made for treatment of injuries received in such sporting activities. Hypocrates had a gymnasium which was roughly equivalent to a physiotherapy department of a modern hospital. Some of the treatments, notably massage and exercise, do not differ materially from those used today. It is believed that the first doctor to receive an official appointment in sports medicine was Galen, who was appointed team physician to the Perganum Gladiators in AD 157.

Some guidelines on the prevention of sports-type injuries

It is obvious that prevention of sports-type injuries is better than cure and many can be prevented by following a few simple rules.

The warm-up

It is important to warm-up before engaging in any sport. This involves stretching all muscle groups with exercises like toe touching, gentle jogging, spot walking, etc. The body is like a motor car – it performs better when warmed. This applies not only to participation in professional athletics, but also in such pleasure pursuits as tennis.

The cool-down

The cool-down (or warm-down) after exercise enables the muscles to revert gradually to their normal function and it assists in the dispersion from the muscle of waste material, in particular urea and lactic acid, built up during the active phase.

Clothing

Most sports have clothes which are particularly designed for them, emphasis being placed on comfort and freedom of movement. Inappropriate clothing can give rise to friction and such conditions as jogger's or runner's nipple can be prevented in the female by the use of properly designed sports bras and in the male by covering the area with a plaster.

Footwear is, of course, very important and the fitting of shoes or boots should be undertaken with a great deal of care.

Rest

In the consideration of preventative measures, rest is of major concern. It is asking for trouble to expect the body to perform well when it is tired and it is in this phase that a large number of injuries take place.

Level of fitness

An individual's level of fitness plays an essential role in the prevention of injury. It must be remembered that the quality of exercise is more important than its quantity. A little regular exercise is more valuable than a large amount taken spasmodically. Two miles jogging or cycling a day, every day, is much better than ten miles on Sunday.

Age factors must also be taken into account. The more vigorous forms of sport, like squash, may be appropriate to younger persons, but exercises such as swimming and walking will certainly be more suitable for older people. Middle-aged people should not undertake jogging before receiving a check-up from their doctor, after which properly cushioned footwear is essential. If possible, the jogging should be done on grass or soft surfaces rather than on concrete. It is advisable to eliminate the competitive spirit, that is not to put a time limit on the covering of a particular circuit, and not to be obsessive. In other words, the body should be listened to, especially when it indicates that abstinence from this form of activity is advisable.

Another valuable form of exercise is provided by exercise bicycles and rowing exercises. With these it is possible to provide suitable programmes for all ages.

First aid

Chapter 19 deals in a general way with this subject, the following problems being particularly associated with sport.

Blisters

Blisters, particularly on the feet, can often be prevented by coating the feet with petroleum jelly (vaseline) or by wearing two pairs of socks. These, of course, should not be of the nylon variety because nylon is non-absorbent.

Abrasions

Abrasions are, of course, a common occurrence and should be treated by washing the area gently with diluted Dettol, TCP or a similar solution, making sure that no particles of dirt remain, because when healing takes place these can leave tattoo-type marks.

Cramp

Cramp is another problem which is often encountered. This is an involuntary shortening of a muscle quite often associated with excessive sweating causing a consequent loss of salt (sodium), or with chilling, for example in swimming. Treatment involves stretching the muscle and firm massage.

> **Remember**
> - No food or drink of any kind should be given to a seriously injured person, because this will delay the effect of anaesthetics in subsequent treatments. In particular, the use of alcohol (such as brandy) should be avoided. Alcohol dilates the surface blood vessels causing loss of heat, so while the patient may feel warmer, the body is getting colder.
> - When dealing with serious injuries, it is important to get the patient to hospital as quickly as possible.
>   - Get someone else to telephone for an ambulance, while you attend the patient.
>   - Move the patient as little as possible, especially in cases of suspected fractures of the spine when the patient should not be moved before medical help arrives. This is important, even if it means stopping the game or activity in progress.

The sports therapist's kit   Some therapists are content with throwing a few useful items in a bag and hoping for the best, the usual result being that the one thing they need is missing. A little careful thought can avoid this contingency. The following list is, therefore, given purely as a guide to which may be added such items as the particular sport determines:

- scissors
- crepe bandage (two-inch)
- one- and two-inch gauze bandages
- triangular bandage
- cotton wool
- sterile gauze pads
- roll of adhesive plaster
- some individual plasters
- smelling salts
- an antiseptic (diluted ready for use)
- petroleum jelly
- tweezers
- aerosol pain killing spray
- crushed ice or cold packs
- disposable gloves
- towel.

ICER   ICER summarises the principles of initial treatment:

- ice
- compression
- elevation
- rest.

These are normally the only methods applied for the first 48 hours after an injury. They should be applied as soon as possible after the injury has taken place because this restricts the development of inflammation and consequently limits oedema in the area.

Ice

Ice packs should not be applied directly to the skin of the area but on top of wet towels or petroleum jelly or oil. This prevents ice burns. Crushed ice is the ideal material, but when this is not available gel bags, having been suitably treated in the refrigerator, or frozen peas, offer reasonable alternatives. When it is necessary to transport these, they should be carried in a thermal bag. If none of the above are available, then towels wrung out in water as cold as is available provide another solution.

Many people feel that the old method of alternating hot and cold water is very effective. This is achieved by having a pail of water as hot as can be reasonably borne and another pail of water as cold as possible.

The area involved is immersed in the cold water for two minutes, taken out and plunged into the hot water for one minute and then back into the cold, repeating for some ten or more minutes. If the area involved is not suitable to be immersed, a similar effect can be achieved by hot and cold towels. When it is necessary and possible the cold treatment may be continued for five minutes in every hour up to a total of 48 hours.

Compression

Compression is normally achieved by firm bandaging or by applying elastic plaster. The aim is to contain the swelling and this requires a certain amount of expertise because the bandaging must not be so tight as to be restrictive of the circulation but it must be firm enough to achieve its object. The method sometimes used is to bandage the area and then to pour cold water over it. This causes the bandage to shrink slightly and therefore tighten up. The advantage of this method is that when the heat of the body has evaporated the water and the bandage begins to stretch again, more water may be poured on, and so on. It is important to practise the art of bandaging and learn spica bandaging, if the opportunity exists. This form of bandaging provides the necessary compression and support without unduly restricting movement.

Elevation

Where possible an injured limb should be elevated so that the blood flows more readily towards the heart. This reduces the pressure caused by fluids in the injured area.

It is generally agreed that cold, compression and elevation are the only desirable treatments for the first 48 hours and during this time the muscle injuries in particular should not be heated, massaged, stretched or electro-stimulated.

Treatments for sports-type injuries

Heat treatments Heat is normally the second stage of the treatment of sports injuries. Heat increases the circulatory flow by dilating the blood vessels and acts as an analgesic by relaxing the muscles

Infrared or radiant heat treatment

For technical information see Chapter 16.

Treatment times are not critical but are normally between 20 and 30 minutes. The heat is directed straight on to the skin – that is, all bandages and plasters must be removed and the skin must be free of oil, creams and embrocation. The lamp should be placed at a distance from the skin where it is comfortably warm but not hot, particular care being taken with diabetic patients who have reduced sensitivity to heat and cold. When treating the face, goggles are not necessary but care should be taken, particularly when the heat is applied near the eye, by removing contact lenses and putting pads of cotton wool over the eyes themselves. This form of treatment may be applied several times a day if necessary.

Paraffin wax treatment

This is the second choice of treatment only because it requires a little more preparation than infrared. It has been used in hospitals for many years because the exterior body can tolerate more heat in this form than in practically any other way. Details of preparation and application are to be found in Chapter 13.

Massage   The mechanical effects of massage include the stretching and mobilising of soft tissues, dispersing all the fluids in the area and stimulating the circulatory system. In addition there is the soothing effect of warm hands over the injured area. All remedial massage must be firm, the pressures being such as to achieve the above objectives but without causing any further damage. Normally remedial or Swedish massage is applied with the use of talc as this allows firm contact without sliding, although sometimes when the area is very painful or swollen, a suitable oil may be used.

The use of massage before involvement in athletic activity can be very useful and it is here that mechanical massagers of the gyratory type can be of particular value. These have a depth effect which is difficult to achieve by hand, together with a speed that cuts down the time considerably, enabling the therapist to treat a much larger number of people.

If massage is given therapeutically it should be accompanied by suitable exercises. These are normally divided into three stages – passive, active and resistive (see Chapter 17).

Faradism   For technical information on Faradism, see Chapter 15.

Faradism is useful because it stimulates the muscles without producing any chemical changes. Faradic current is very similar to the form of energy which flows down a motor nerve and is used for the same effect, that is to operate the muscle. It is, therefore, a passive form of exercise, the speed and power both being regulated by the therapist. In this way it is possible to increase the tonus of a muscle to speed up its rehabilitation.

Most modern instruments are equipped with variable surge speed and controllable power. The surge speed indicates the number of times the muscle is activated and this can vary between, say, five times a minute and 100 times a minute. Very weak or debilitated muscles are normally worked at the very slow speeds and the rate increased as the muscle improves to a normal maximum of 50–60 movements per minute.

Generally, Faradism is used once a day. In special circumstances, it can be applied two or three times. Faradism may also be used for muscle prognosis, thus determining whether the muscle is improving or retrograding under treatment. For this purpose special electrodes are used, not the normal pads which are usually supplied with Faradic instruments, and the amount of current required to move the muscle is measured. If more current than previously is needed to move the muscle, it is retrogressing, whilst if less current is used then it is improving. Such a measurement, of course, requires accurate knowledge of the origin and insertion of the muscle concerned.

There are many multi-output instruments available, but these are rarely necessary for the sports therapist; a small instrument having two or four outputs is all that is required. If the instrument is only to be used in a static situation then the choice will obviously be a mains instrument, the battery-operated type being the choice of the visiting practitioner.

Normally faradic treatment may only be applied after consultation with the patient's doctor.

Vacuum suction   This is dealt with in detail in Chapter 14.

Although many people associate vacuum suction with slimming techniques, its use for this purpose is of reasonably recent origin, suction cups having been used for thousands of years for their therapeutic value.

The therapeutic effects of vacuum suction include an increased blood and lymph flow, stimulated metabolism and the production of a satisfactory hyperaemia. It has been used successfully for muscle toning, post-traumatic circulatory disorders and has proved particularly valuable in the reduction of oedema. As a treatment form it can prove invaluable for such conditions as bursitis, synovitis, epicondylitis and all those inflammatory conditions which are accompanied by oedema. In working over painful areas a very low vacuum should be used, say 5 per cent, gradually increasing to a maximum of not more than 15 per cent when pain has completely disappeared. Treatment is accelerated when the area has been previously heated, for example, with a radiant heat lamp. To be effective, treatment should be applied once a day.

Sterilising procedures

It is appreciated that sterilising procedures are very difficult on the sports field but, on returning to the centre, all items which have been used should be suitably treated:

- Scissors and tweezers should be immersed in surgical spirit or a strong solution of Dettol.
- Disposable items should preferably be burned and other items such as gel bags should be thoroughly cleaned with antiseptic solution.
- Any items which have been used out of the therapist's sports kit should be replaced so that it is ready for immediate use.

21 Ultrasound and its Use in Treatment

Ultrasound means 'beyond sound', i.e. frequencies beyond normal audible range. Ultrasound, or ultrasonic, waves have a number of varied uses, including cleaning metal, underwater echo sounding, medical diagnosis (particularly in pregnancy), as well as physical therapy.

Production of ultrasonic waves

Ultrasonic waves are not part of the electromagnetic spectrum in the way that short waves or microwaves are. Although they are electrically produced, ultrasonic waves are compression waves.

The phenomenon of an aircraft breaking through the 'sound barrier' is well known to most people, though not everyone understands exactly what happens. An aircraft in flight produces a lot of noise and this noise travels ahead of it at speeds that vary with the height of the aircraft. Assume that an aircraft is travelling at 500 miles per hour at a height at which the sound waves that it produces travel at 650 miles per hour. The sound waves will be travelling 150 miles per hour faster than the aircraft so there is no possibility of the aircraft overtaking them. However, when the aircraft exceeds 650 miles per hour, it will catch up with and pass through the sound waves which it has itself produced. These compressed waves form an almost solid wall which the aircraft pushes aside as it passes through, causing the first crack noise that we hear when an aircraft passes through the 'sound barrier'. After the aircraft has passed through the waves they join together again causing the second crack noise. Designers of supersonic planes are therefore very concerned not only with ensuring that the strength of the aircraft is sufficient to allow it to pass through the sound waves, but also that the aircraft will produce as little resistance as possible in breaking the sound waves apart.

If a rod of ferro-electric metal is magnetised by means of an electric current, one end becomes the north pole and the other becomes the south pole. The north and south poles attract each other, so the rod will become fractionally shorter when the current passes. If the applied current is switched rapidly on and off, greater alteration in the length of the rod is produced. In other words the rod will be vibrating, and the vibrations will produce waves of sound. When the same principle is applied to a suitably cut quartz crystal, it will vibrate at very high speeds and so produce ultrasound.

176

In contrast to electromagnetic radiation, for example, ultrasound is not able to travel in a vacuum. Its speed through different materials varies considerably as is shown by the following approximate travel speeds:

- air   300 metres per second
- fresh water   1400 metres per second
- sea water   1500 metres per second
- muscular tissue   1400 metres per second
- fatty tissue   1600 metres per second.

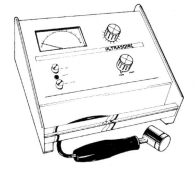

ULTRASOUND TREATMENT UNIT

In the early ultrasound machines the current applied to the crystal face was generated by means of valves and this, combined with the type of mounting used for the crystal in the very large heads used at that time, involved the production of a good deal of heat which meant that the head had to be watercooled. The early instruments were very large (about the size of a small desk) and could only be operated on a site where running water was readily available. Most of these problems have now been overcome – modern instruments are transistorised and the heads are very much smaller so that cooling is no longer necessary and the instruments themselves are very compact and portable.

Some confusion is created by instruments advertised as 'audio-sonic', i.e. sound producing. These small units are percussors and not in any way related to the instruments described in this chapter.

The effects of ultrasound

It is generally agreed that ultrasound energy applied to the human body has four types of effect:

- mechanical
- chemical or biological
- thermal
- neural.

Mechanical effects

The main mechanical effect is really micro-massage. Massage as a form of physical medicine has been used for very many centuries – certainly since the days of Hippocrates and probably earlier. Massage in general terms exerts a series of pressures on the body tissue and then releases them, thus relaxing the tissue.

As has already been seen, ultrasound also produces pressures and when these are applied to the human body they compress and release the tissue as in massage but at very much faster speeds. Also, because of the speed, they are able to effect a micro-massage on tissue which would not produce a response to hand massage. Additionally, because of the controllability of the energy, it is possible to apply ultrasonic massage to areas which would be too painful for hand massage.

Another effect of these very fast sound waves is the oscillation of particles within the energy field. This is generally believed to improve the blood circulation and lymphatic drainage of the site treated, as well as loosening or disintegrating granules associated with rheumatic conditions.

Chemical or biological effects There are a number of chemical effects created by ultrasound waves and it is not the purpose of this chapter to go into these in detail. It will therefore be sufficient to list the more measurable biological reactions so that those who are interested in such physiological effects will be acquainted with the primary processes involved. It has been noted that the following chemical effects can be attributed to ultrasound irradiation:

- improved permeability of all membranes to sodium and potassium ions
- inhibition of inflammatory processes
- vaso dilation
- analgesia
- a change of tissue pH
- liberation of homochronologically active materials – transport of ions (see the section on phonophoresis later in this chapter)
- improved hyperaemia.

Thermal effects The thermal, or heat, effect of ultrasound waves is really a by-product, but none the less a very important one. The heat is produced by the friction created by the waves passing through the tissue. The advantage of this form of thermal activity against others in common use is that it is target heat. Infrared, short wave and microwave treatments have a more general heating effect on the whole of an area whereas ultrasound may be directed at the lesion itself.

Neural effects It is a well known fact that the nervous system responds readily to external stimuli as shown by the effects of galvanism, Faradism, etc. The treatment of the nervous system, and in particular the treatment of autonomic processes, with ultrasound waves is in its infancy and it is not the purpose of this chapter to explain how neural effects are achieved, but it would appear that ultrasound waves are stimulating or exciting to the processes involved. As described in Chapter 6, the autonomic system has two branches – the sympathetic and the para-sympathetic – and irradiation of the corresponding segments and spinal nerve roots produce somewhat different results:

- stimulation of the sympathetic system raises blood pressure and blood sugar level, causes sweating and excites secretion of adrenalin
- stimulation of the para-sympathetic system retards the heart, promotes secretion of insulin and lowers blood sugar level.

In arriving at a conclusion as to how the excitation actually takes place it is well worth considering a hypothesis based on the discoveries of Professor Eiichifukada of Tokyo University. He reports that large

178

molecules such as protein or cellulose exhibit the piezoelectric effect when subjected to pressure. This produces electric charges on their surfaces and it could be that sound pressure produced by ultrasound waves causes the large molecules to develop a piezoelectric charge which, in turn, stimulates nerves as well as muscles.

Although the four types of effect of ultrasound irradiation are described separately above, this is not intended to suggest that they are independent in action. Experience shows that a combination of each of the four effects is involved in most of the cures or improvements attributed to ultrasound treatment.

Methods of application

Early ultrasound instruments were equipped with very large heads delivering, in many cases, a great deal of power. This resulted not only in unnecessary heat but sometimes in unpleasant side-effects because of the destructive nature of the high energy used. However, much research and experience has shown that a safe maximum wattage is 3 W/cm^2 delivered to a head of 5 cm^2. This gives a total usable energy of 15 W though, as will be seen later, this maximum is rarely used. However, this is considered to be a safe maximum, subject of course, as in all physical treatments, to such warning signals as pain.

As has already been seen, ultrasound waves are largely ineffective in air as they travel slowly through this medium, but they do travel well through water and body tissue. It is particularly important, therefore, that there should be no air space between the treatment head and the body. For this purpose, the site to be treated is covered with a suitable coupling material to enable the head not only to move easily but also to eliminate air. Sometimes liquid paraffin or a massage oil is used as a coupling material. This has, of course, good viscosity and allows the head to travel easily but because of its lack of bulk it does not fill up all the cracks and spaces on the surface of the body and is, therefore, not an ideal coupling material. Most manufacturers sell a cream or gel which is comparatively inexpensive and has been especially designed for the coupling purpose.

SOUND HEAD WITHOUT COUPLING
MATERIAL – AIR SPACE PRESENT

SOUND HEAD WITH COUPLING
MATERIAL – AIR SPACE ELIMINATED

A very satisfactory method of treating uneven surfaces such as feet and hands is the water bath method. Here the extremity is placed in a bath of water, a Schnee bath or similar, and the treatment head is also placed in the water and directed at the lesion site. The distance between the head and the skin can be up to 10 cm although it is more

179

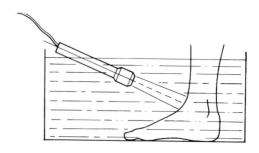

A WATER BATH

usual to keep the head about 2 cm away from the treatment area. Care should be taken to avoid direct contact between the head and the skin under water. When warm tap water is used in the bath, air bubbles will separate out after a short while and adhere to the skin and the treatment head. As ultrasound does not travel well through air, these bubbles will impede treatment and they should be removed. If purified or well-boiled water is used this procedure becomes unnecessary.

Whilst the water bath method is suitable for the extremities, the irregular shape of the spine also requires special consideration. It is not normally possible to immerse the whole of the spine in water when giving treatment, so a coupling cushion is involved. The coupling cushion is made of plastic film or thin rubber and filled with degassed water to at least 80–90 per cent of the bag's capacity, enabling it to be moulded to the part to be treated. The part is then covered with the normal coupling cream and the coupling cushion is put in position and held there by two fingers of the therapist's hand. The upper surface of the cushion is then covered with cream and the head of the ultrasonic unit is applied to this and used in the ordinary way.

Most instruments are now supplied with two modes of operation:

- *continuous mode*, where the current is continuous and uninterrupted
- *pulsed mode*, where the energy is pulsed in periods stated by the manufacturers, such as one on – one off, or one on – four off. In the latter, for every 10 min of operation, the energy would be on for 2 min and off for 8 min.

Pulsed energy is particularly valuable for treating recent injuries where periostal pain might become intolerable if the current was applied continuously. Many therapists, however, prefer to use continuous current on old, established lesions because they argue that the normal method of contact treatment, which is to move the head in small circles, has the effect of interrupting the energy over any particular point. The pulsed mode should, however, be used in all those cases where it is important that there should be no build up of heat, because the rest period between the bursts of output enables the circulation to cool the area.

Choice of frequency   It is important to remember that the higher the frequency, the smaller the depth of penetration. So, conversely, the lower the frequency, within certain limits, the higher the depth of penetration. It should be emphasised that there is no apparent difference in the effect of the treatment when given with, say, 1 MHz or 3 MHz. The only difference is to be found in the depth of penetration. An ultrasonic beam does not terminate, it goes on with ever decreasing power in much the same way as a light beam does. In ultrasound treatment the energy is considered to have lost most of its effectiveness when the tissue through which it is passed reduces its power to half. Without going into the more complicated physics involved in these measurements, it is approximately correct to say that for the same power or energy output, 3 MHz only effectively penetrates about one third of the distance that 1 MHz does. With the same power, 1 MHz would penetrate to a depth of 5 cm compared with about 1.4 cm penetration with 3 MHz. Because of this, most manufacturers have now concentrated on the production of instruments which operate at or around 1 MHz. A few manufacturers provide the alternative frequency of 3 MHz, particularly for the benefit of people who specialise in treatment of the skin or the immediate subcutaneous tissue, where depth effect is not so important.

As mentioned earlier, most instruments now are designed to deliver a maximum of 3 W/cm^2 and they are all fitted with control knobs which give a selection of power outputs varying from as low as 0.1 W/cm^2 to the maximum of 3 W/cm^2. You will quickly find the power output which is the most suitable for your speciality. It is normally considered wise to operate at somewhere between 1 and 1.5 W/cm^2.

Treatment indications

It is not the purpose of this chapter, nor is it possible, to provide a complete list of all the conditions which can be treated by ultrasound. The Erlangen Ultrasonic Conference in 1949 reviewed over 100 000 treatments and since then much water has flowed under the bridge. Many more cases and types of case will be on file as having received beneficial effects from *insonation*. Some guidelines, however, are obviously of value and the table of conditions on page 182, giving treatment times and the amount of energy used, should give you a reasonably accurate idea of the range of conditions for which this form of treatment is suitable.

It is now generally accepted that in all cases of trauma where physical medicine would normally be indicated, ultrasonic therapy may be applied immediately after the trauma has occurred. This stimulates the absorption of oedema and starts a cycle around the injured structures which reduces pain, decreases muscle spasm and this, in turn, further reduces the pain level. Normal movements can be performed almost at once, resulting in minimal residual waste products and ensuring that a very low level of fibrous tissue is laid down. This applies especially to severe sprains and strains of muscle fibres, tendons and ligaments, dislocations and fractures, acute tenosynovitis, tendinitis, synovitis and capsulitis. In all these conditions pulsed ultrasound is indicated because of the possible high pain level.

Ultrasound treatment of selected conditions

Condition	Ultrasound treatment			
	Intensity	Mode	Duration	Note
Traumatic synovitis	0.75–1.00 W	Pulse	3 min	Twice daily
Ligament injuries	1.00–1.25 W	Continuous	Up to 5 min	Every other day
Contusions	1.00–1.25 W	Continuous	5 min	Twice on day of injury, once a day thereafter
Sprains, strains	1.00 W	Pulse or continuous	5 min	Twice daily; choose pulse or continuous according to pain level
Metasalgia	1.00–1.25 W	Continuous	5 min	In water bath
Torn muscles or ligaments	1.00 W	Pulse or continuous	5 min	Twice on day of injury, once a day thereafter
Fractures where the splints are removable	1.00 W	Pulse	5 min	Daily
Frozen shoulder	1.00–1.50 W	Pulse or continuous	3 min	Every other day
Fibrositis	1.00–1.50 W	Continuous	5 min	Every other day
Rheumatoid arthritis	1.00 W	Continuous	3 min	Twice a week
Brachial neuritis	0.75–1.00 W	Continuous	5 min	Daily
Sciatic neuritis	1.00 W	Pulse	2 min	Daily
Bronchial asthma	1.00–1.50 W	Continuous	2 min	Along subclavian stellate ganglion
Keloids	1.50 W	Continuous	5 min	Twice a week
Herpes zosta	1.00 W	Pulse or continuous	3 min	Every other day
Bursitis	1.00 W	Pulse or continuous	3 min	Daily

Contra-indications to ultrasound treatment

For the instrument The energy should not be switched on until you are ready to use the instrument, that is when the treatment head is either in contact with the patient or in a water bath. Allowing the treatment head to operate in free air for any length of time is likely to result in damage.

For the patient   The following contra-indications are given purely as a guide. Many authorities differ considerably on what they consider to be dangerous uses of ultrasound. For example, while the majority would not use sound waves over the heart, there are some who use them specifically to treat heart conditions. As the maxim 'if in doubt – don't' is particularly applicable to physical medicine, the following list of contra-indications may be considered unless or until experience and increased knowledge invalidates them.

Ultrasound treatment is contra-indicated:

- over the cardiac region
- in cardio-vascular conditions such as thrombosis and phlebitis
- over the brain
- over the eyes
- over the reproductive organs
- over the abdomen, especially in the case of pregnant women because of the risk of abortion
- over tumours, whether benign or malignant
- in cases of acute sepsis
- in cases of acute inflammation, e.g. osteomyelitis
- over carbuncles or boils
- in cases of pulmonary or bone tuberculosis
- on patients suffering from haemophilia or hyperthyroidism.

No patient should continue to receive ultrasound treatment at the same energy level after complaining of excess heat, a burning sensation or pain. This indicates that the upper limits of tolerance have been reached and the treatment should be immediately modified – that is, the energy should be reduced to a point where these reactions do not re-occur.

Phonophoresis

Phonophoresis is one of the very valuable treatments available with ultrasound, but its use developed slowly. Although early work was done in this field by the Germans it was, to an extent, neglected in favour of the more usual physiotherapy type of treatment.

Reference has already been made in this book (page 143) to iontophoresis or ionisation by means of a galvanic current. This causes charged particles to move along a path from one electrode to the other, but electrically neutral particles are not affected. The limitation of this form of treatment is that only certain substances (those carrying positive or negative charges) can effectively be introduced into the system.

Ultrasound does not suffer from these disadvantages because, being non-electrical, it does not dissociate the molecule in any way. By its sheer unidirectional power it is able to force the whole molecule into the tissue, and this process is known as *phonophoresis*. There is no way in which it is possible to introduce the whole molecule into the system using electrophoresis.

In addition to its medical uses, beauty therapists have found this method of considerable value when they wish to introduce beauty preparations into subcutaneous tissue. As a general guide, for subcutaneous treatments an intensity of 0.75–1.00 W and a treatment time of about five minutes should be sufficient. For joints and deep-seated penetration, a higher intensity will be needed and this should be pulsed in order to prevent a heat build-up in the tissue which could, in certain circumstances, interfere with the treatment.

Other uses of ultrasound

Some of the other uses of ultrasound are commercial, others are of defence value or of use in science and perhaps especially in medicine – that is, general medicine or surgery, as opposed to physical medicine which has been dealt with in the previous chapters.

The speed of the agitations made possible by ultrasound equipment means that it is used extensively by pharmaceutical and chemical companies for mixing paints and other materials. Sonar equipment, as used by the navy for detecting underwater objects such as submarines, is very well known. It is also used for detecting faults in the metal plates of ships and metal fatigue in aircraft. Ultrasound has also been used to clean clothes, the dirt particles being vibrated out of the fibres, thus avoiding the need for the chemicals used in normal dry cleaning.

The other particular value which ultrasound has in medicine is in *sonography*. This is the use of ultrasound energy to take 'photographs' of the interior of the body, in much the same way that X-rays are used, but without some of the damaging effects which are associated with X-rays. This is particularly of value in determining the exact position of, for example, a baby in the womb – diagnosis which medicine has been reluctant in the past to achieve with X-rays because of the possible damage to the baby. The ultrasound method is now widely used in maternity departments and enables doctors to study actual pictures of the baby's beating heart before it is born and also to locate malignancies or deformities. This means that the necessary medical action can be taken. The technique is completely painless and has no harmful effects on either mother or baby.

22 The Role of Massage in Stress Management

It is generally accepted that modern living can be very stressful. It is important to understand the causes of stress, to differentiate between good and bad stress, and how massage contributes to its management.

Stress

Not all stress is harmful. Many people do their best work when stressed. The need to achieve and the drive to obtain success can in themselves be helpful rather than harmful factors and may contribute to a harmonious lifestyle. Much outstanding work in the fields of science, arts and business has been attained under conditions of stress. Therefore it is necessary to look at stress, its causes and the factors which can make it harmful.

Death from heart attacks and coronary artery disease is often associated with over-achieving, high-flying executives, but this is not necessarily so. In a study of the civil service (The Whitehall Study) over a ten-year period, it was found that death rates from coronary disease were lowest in the administrative grades and highest in the lowest grade. The researchers found that people on higher grades felt more in control of their work and better supported by friends and colleagues so that, although their lives appeared more stressful, they were able to cope. These people had more hobbies and interests outside work. Whilst not suggesting that stress or the lack of it was the only factor contributing to these deaths during working life, it must be assumed that it played an important part. Other studies have confirmed that people who are employed in positions where they have job satisfaction and enjoy a certain amount of control have a better health record. For example, a review carried out by the Medical Officer of the British Institute of Directors showed that chairpersons of companies rarely suffer heart attacks whilst in office.

We will see later that stress manifests itself in many different ways, but it originated in antiquity. The fight or flight syndrome was seen in our ancestors who, when faced by marauding enemies or wild animals, had only two choices – either to stay and fight or to run away. Both choices required an increase in energy which the body provided through release of adrenalin.

In modern life we are not very likely to be faced with these alternatives, but we may still feel angry because of a very difficult customer, or fear when (unjustifiably) we are 'put on the carpet' by our boss, or frustrated by non-recognition of our work. In these circumstances, adrenalin is released but, because we are unable to use it (i.e. to fight), it remains as a harmful substance in the body. One of the effects of this is a chemical reaction with 'good' cholesterol converting it to 'bad' cholesterol. This, in turn, causes a hard waxy substance to build up on the inner walls of arteries, the reduced bore of the blood vessels increasing the blood pressure, or hypertension. In some large Japanese companies they have rubber models of bosses in the company's gymnasium so that, having to stand and take a telling off by the boss, they may later visit the gymnasium and knock the 'living daylights' out of the rubber model! It has been found that this using up of the adrenalin has a profound effect in restoring normality to the situation.

It is useful to look at the physiological pathway of fear and anger:

- *fear* causes an increase of adrenalin
- *anger* causes an increase of noradrenalin.

Together they equip us for emergency action. They contract the arteries; the heart beats faster to supply more blood which is drawn back from the skin in order to make more available. In addition, the blood clotting time is quickened and the liver is stimulated to release more glycogen for muscle energy. The chart opposite shows the pathway.

The pituitary gland has two lobes:

- the *anterior lobe*, which secretes:
    - adrenocorticotropic hormone – adrenals
    - thyrotropic hormone – which regulates the thyroid
    - somatropic hormone – which regulate growth
    - gonadotropic hormone – sex
- the *posterior lobe*, which secretes:
    - oxytocin – uterine muscles and mammary glands
    - vasopressin – muscles – blood pressure.

In a healthy body all these hormones are balanced, but when one of them is over-produced, as in harmful stress, disease can result.

Body physiology requires time to adjust to environmental changes and the following timetable shows why we currently have problems:

- in the Stone Age humans had 10 000 years to adjust
- in the Bronze Age they had 1000 years to adjust
- in the Iron Age they had 100 years
- In our age we have had 50 years to adjust to nuclear energy and molecular biology, and 20 years to adjust to genetic engineering and lap-top computers.

The speed of change has been accompanied by a number of other factors which contribute to stress:

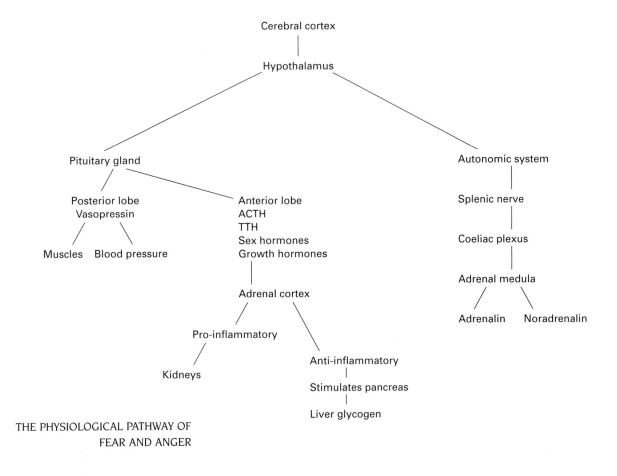

THE PHYSIOLOGICAL PATHWAY OF
FEAR AND ANGER

- *a lifestyle of constantly meeting deadlines/constant hurry*
- *noise* In a service test, 75 per cent of soldiers who had been subjected to high noise level (9 dc) doubled their margin of visual error for one hour afterwards.
- *frustration* Experiments on rats showed deformation of adrenals, thyroids, hearts and lungs.
- *pollution* and its effects especially on the respiratory system
- *increasing number of cars* which combine the four factors above.

Medical symptoms of stress Harmful stress shows itself in a number of medical symptoms: apprehension, generalised feelings of anxiety, tense headaches, unusual fatigue, frigidity, impotence, poor concentration, decreasing ability to make decisions, hyperventilation, increased irritability, eating/drinking/smoking too much.

Types of stress There are three fundamental stresses:

- *mortal combat* Today films, videos and TV keep the idea alive.
- *fight for survival* Today it is to keep up with the Jones's – or overtake them.
- *fear of death* This appears to be more obvious today with the decreasing role of religion.

187

Characteristics of stress   There are three elements involved in stress:

- *psychological*, e.g. a feeling of inadequacy or inferiority
- *physical*, e.g. tension in muscles of neck and shoulders
- *emotional*, e.g. hate and love/guilt.

Stressed persons normally experience at least two of these and more often all three.

Causes of stress   Stressors, things which causes stress, may be:

- *environmental*, such as unsuitable working conditions, hunched over a computer or word processor
- *chemical*, such as working in a smoke or other polluted atmosphere
- *workload-related*, such as pressure to complete on time.
- *financial*.

Measurement of stress   Psychologists have evaluated the stress effect of life events. The most widely used method being the Holmes-Rahe scale (see opposite).

If a person's total score adds up to between 150 and 400 over a 12-month period, there is indication of developing some stress-related illness unless care is taken. A score of over 400 indicates some evidence of stress-related illness being present (see the list of medical symptoms on page 187). This scale is obviously only a guide, but if taken seriously it can be used as an indicator of preventative treatment.

Treatment of stress

Non-medical treatment includes:

- *better control of working life, including*:
  - leaving earlier for the office, train or plane so that if there is an unexpected hold-up, you have a margin of time
  - planning and prioritising each day's activities
  - not setting targets or deadlines that are unreasonable
  - finishing one task before another is undertaken
  - learning to delegate – no one is indispensable
  - allowing time for meal breaks, rather than eating or drinking whilst still working.
- *using leisure time more effectively by*:
  - reserving time for leisure activities
  - including time each day for active exercise, whether it be in a gym, jogging (for younger people), walking or swimming (for older people)
  - having a creative rather than competitive hobby, e.g. painting, photography or music.

The Holmes-Rahe scale — Life event	Lifechange units
Death of spouse	100
Divorce	73
Marital separation	65
Imprisonment	63
Death of close family member	63
Personal injury or illness	53
Marriage	50
Dismissal from work	47
Marital reconciliation	45
Retirement	45
Change in health of family member	44
Pregnancy	40
Sexual difficulties	39
Gain a new family member	39
Business readjustment	39
Change in financial state	38
Change in number of arguments with spouse	35
Major mortgage	32
Foreclosure of mortgage or loan	30
Change in responsibilities at work	29
Son or daughter leaving home	29
Trouble with in-laws	29
Outstanding personal achievement	28
Spouse begins or stops work	26
Begin or end school	26
Change in living conditions	25
Revision of personal habits	24
Trouble with boss	23
Change in work hours or conditions	20
Change in residence	20
Change in schools	20
Change in recreation	19
Change in church activities	19
Change in social activities	18
Minor mortgage or loan	17
Change in sleeping habits	16
Change in number of family reunions	15
Change in eating habits	15
Vacation	13
Christmas	12
Minor violation of the law	11

- *touch treatment (massage) by a professional or a sympathetic friend*
  Touch in the form of massage is a powerful tool in treating or preventing stress. In a research project, Harvard Medical School patients about to have an operation were divided into two groups. The anaesthetist visited the first group and carefully explained the procedure. He did the same for the second group except that in addition he sat on the bed of each patient for around five minutes holding their hand and being generally warm and sympathetic. After the operations the second group required only half the amount of drugs on average and were discharged three days earlier.

Massage Accepting that massage *is* an appropriate treatment, the question then arises as to the more suitable type – whole body or localised? When time and money allow, the choice must be the whole body holistic massage, preferably with aromatic oils applied by an aroma-therapist. The alternative, localised massage, is however also very effective.

Most physical stress or tension is exhibited in the back, shoulders and neck, together with the hands and arms of office workers, especially those operating mechanical devices.

The following is a programme which can easily be applied in the workplace. It requires a minimum of equipment and is not time-consuming – an average of 15 minutes per client being reasonable. The massage is normally scheduled for the workplace of the client to reduce interference with work.

Massage, which consists mainly of effleurage, pétrissage and kneading, is normally confined to:

- fingers, hands and lower arms
- shoulders and upper spine
- neck up to the base of the skull.

Sometimes scalp massage may be included, in which case the treatment lasts, say, 20 minutes.

Undressing is kept to a minimum, leaving the shoulders bare and most of the upper body being wrapped in a large towel. The client will be seated on his or her own chair though the opposite way round in order to provide easy access to shoulders and neck.

The following equipment is required, which can be carried easily in a holdall:

- a large towel
- talc and oil – to client's choice
- tissues
- cologne, in case oil (not aromatic) is used.

The physical effect of this treatment on machine operators is very good and increased output more than compensates for the time taken. The psychological and physical effect on all participants results in reduced fatigue, improved output and better relationships with colleagues.

A number of large companies encourage their employees to participate in programmes of massage in the workplace, but there is tremendous scope for further development. Obviously permission has to be obtained from the management first, and decisions need to be made about the frequency of visits, which sections will take part and who will pay – the client or the company. A very good argument can be made for the company to pay, because it will be the beneficiary of more efficient, happier employees.

A questionnaire sent out to all employed persons at a UK hospice asked whether they felt a massage would be helpful to them in their work and if so which type. Seventy per cent of the questionnaires were returned – 47 per cent from nurses, 19 per cent from domestic staff (porters, caterers), 19 per cent from clerical staff and 16 per cent from others (including other professionals). The results were as follows – with a certain amount of overlap:

- for full body massage – 10 per cent
- for shoulder and neck massage – 81 per cent
- for hand massage – 23 per cent
- for scalp massage – 38 per cent
- for foot massage – 23 per cent.

Some additional aids to stress control

- Smile and respond positively to others.
- Avoid hostility.
- Take time to look at your own values and destination.
- Develop a sense of fun and an ability to laugh at yourself.
- Avoid sameness and lack of change.
- Do something for others without hope of reward.
- Concentrate on what is worth doing, rather than worth having.

And finally, two quotations which sum it all up:

'Volumes are now written and spoken about the effect of the mind on the body. Much of it is true but I wish a little more was taught on the effect of the body on the mind.'

Florence Nightingale in 1859

'Teach him to live rather than avoid death. Life is not breath but action, the use of our senses, mind, faculties, every part of ourselves which makes us conscious of our being.'

Jean Jacques Rousseau

i.e. to enjoy life is the best way to lengthen it.

23 Nutrition: A General Introduction

CONTRIBUTED BY PAUL GODWIN

Why do we need to study nutrition? 'We all know that the majority of people develop and remain in good health provided they get enough to eat.' This statement is not true – many people who appear to eat enough food are clinically malnourished, and recent studies of the elderly maintain that as many as 40 per cent are suffering from malnutrition, although they are eating regular meals. At the other end of the scale, in 1992 two university teams researching the difference between the levels of IQ in various children found, under double blind trials, that they could improve their non-verbal reasoning scores by between seven and 20 points by improving their vitamin and mineral input by direct supplementation on a daily basis. Here we have two well researched studies which suggest that 'getting enough to eat' is not enough. The general adult population must also have nutritional problems, but their plight has so far, by and large, gone unresearched, except in certain specific areas where funds are made available by government or industry.

Do we understand what our foods provide for us? How they are broken down and used by the body? How they are used to protect us from disease processes? Do we know how they can heal us when we suffer from infections of various types? Do we know enough about the quality and freshness of the food we eat? Do we understand enough about the processing of our foods? A comprehensive understanding of the nutrients which make up our diet, and the way in which they are processed and used by the human body is the science of nutrition.

Nutrients

Nutrients present in our food chain are many and varied, but fall into the following main categories:

- water
- proteins
- carbohydrates
- fats
- vitamins
- minerals.

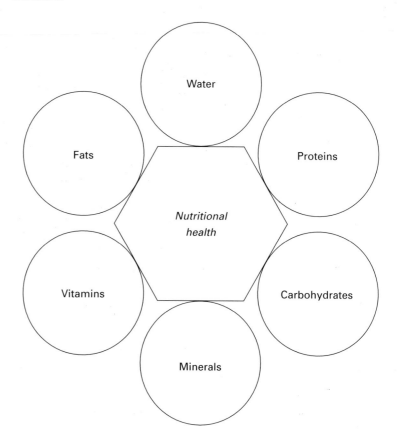

THE HEXAGRAM OF NUTRITIONAL HEALTH, SHOWING THE SIX ESSENTIAL NUTRIENTS

Water Water is the most important nutrient. When you consider that the adult body weight is approximately 60 per cent water, and an infant's body weight can be as much as 70 per cent water, you can see that a loss of 20 per cent of body fluids can cause serious malfunction or death.

Water is the main constituent of all body fluids including blood, lymph, urine and perspiration. It is important in regulating the acid/alkaline balance, the movement of nutrients around the body and the flow of electrolytic solutions which are so important in the operation of the nervous system. Water is a compound of hydrogen and oxygen (H_2O).

Water has been described as the 'staff of life without which we perish'; we can exist without food for some months, but we can only be without water for a few days before we die. Current thinking on water intake for a healthy life is approximately 1½ litres of pure water a day, not including beverages and food products which contain water.

Protein

The word protein comes from the Greek, *proto*, meaning first and, after water, protein is the most plentiful substance in the body. Protein in food is broken down into *amino acids* during the digestive process and these are used in the vital construction, growth and maintenance of every tissue in the body. It is also essential for the production of hormones, infection-fighting antibodies and enzymes, but any excess is used as a source of instant energy or is laid down as fat. All proteins are compounds of carbon, hydrogen, oxygen and nitrogen, together with a variety of minerals and trace elements.

There are approximately 20 amino acids and they are divided into:

- eight *essential amino acids*, which cannot be produced by the body and therefore have to come from food
- 12 *non-essential amino acids*, which are produced in the body from excess essential amino acids in the diet.

Excess amino acids cannot be stored in the body, and so a balanced assortment of proteins containing the required essential amino acids needs to be part of the daily diet.

Excess protein intake can be dangerous for the body because it has to be processed. Surplus nitrogen-carrying amino acids are processed in the liver and turned into urea, which is passed to the kidneys and excreted as urine. All other surplus amino acids are converted to glucose which can be used as an immediate source of energy, or laid down as fat.

Dietary sources of protein are:

- meat
- fish and shellfish
- dairy products
- eggs
- grains and pulses.

Carbohydrates

There are three types of carbohydrate in food:

- *sugars*
- *starches*
- *cellulose*, including *dietary fibre*.

Carbohydrates are compounds formed from carbon, hydrogen, oxygen, water, minerals and other trace elements.

Dietary carbohydrates are the body's preferred primary *energy* source for all body functions, although fats and proteins can be converted to energy when required.

A variety of different sugars are broken down in the digestive system and enter the blood stream where they trigger the release of *insulin* from the pancreas. Insulin is a hormone which converts sugar into glycogen. Glycogen is actually a polysaccharide (many sugars) which cannot be used by the body for immediate energy needs, but can be stored for later processing. It is stored in the muscles and liver, and when energy is required the hormone *adrenalin* is released from the adrenal glands and converts the glycogen back to sugars for use as energy.

Some sugars are not converted to glycogen, but are used for the body's immediate energy needs.

Carbohydrates can be classified in four groups:

- *monosaccharides* (simple sugars), including glucose, fructose and galactose
- *disaccharides* (two monosaccharides minus water), including sucrose, maltose and lactose
- *polysaccharides* (complex compounds), including starches, dextrins and glycogen (synthesised in liver and muscle from glucose)
- *indigestible polysaccharides* (various forms of dietary fibre), including cellulose, lignin and pectin.

Dietary sources of carbohydrates are:

- *sugars*, from cane and beet sugar, honey, natural fruit sugars, molasses
- *starches*, from whole grains, pulses (legumes), vegetables, fruit
- *cellulose*, including fibre and pectin, from whole grains, pulses (legumes), vegetables, fruit.

Fats

Fats (Lipids) have recently been targeted as the main cause of coronary heart disease, and we have all been told that we have to reduce the fats in our diet to maintain health. While this is perfectly true, it must also be remembered that fats are essential to our well-being, and that moderate consumption of the right kind of fats will bring us energy and health. Like carbohydrates, fats are compounds of carbon, hydrogen and oxygen, but the proportion of oxygen is much lower. The common property of all fats is their insolubility in water.

Fat supplies energy more economically than any other nutrient, but must first be stored before it can be used. So although it provides a concentrated source, it is not a quick source of energy like sugar, which can enter the bloodstream in minutes. Fat takes between three and six hours after it has been eaten before it can be utilised.

In chemical terms, the fat in our foods consists mainly of mixtures of triglycerides. Each triglyceride is a combination of three *fatty acids* of various kinds and glycerol, bound together in a system of double bonds. Many fatty acids are present in nature and they are constituents of most of our foods. There are different types of fatty acids:

- *saturated fatty acids*, which have no double bonds and are therefore very stable, such as lard, suet and cocoa butter
- *unsaturated fatty acids*, which may be either:

- *monounsaturated*, which have only one double bond and provide the bulk of most fats, especially olive oil where they make up 70 per cent of the total fatty acid content

- *polyunsaturated*, which contain various numbers of double bonds and are very unstable and often turn to liquid.

Two unsaturated fatty acids in particular are known as *essential fatty acids* because they are essential for growth but cannot be manufactured in the body. These are:

- *linoleic acid*, which is found in abundance in vegetable seed oils, such as sunflower oil, corn oil and soya oil, and is present in small concentrations in some animal fats, such as pork

- *linolenic acid*, which occurs in small amounts in some vegetable oils such as linseed oil.

These need to be included in small quantities in the diet for normal health.

A third unsaturated fatty acid, *arachidonic acid*, is synthesised in the body when adequate supplies of linoleic acid are present.

Vitamins

Vitamins are naturally occurring *organic substances* which cannot be synthesised within the body, but are essential, in regulated amounts, to the maintenance and health of every tissue in the body. Vitamins are obtained from various food sources, but some vitamins are input to the digestive system in their *provitamin* or precursor form and are converted within the body to the required vitamin.

Vitamins may be:

- *water-soluble* – vitamins B and C
- *fat-soluble* – vitamins A, D, E and K.

Excessive dietary intake of water-soluble vitamins is relatively harmless because any excess is excreted in urine. However, excessive intake of fat-soluble vitamins may be dangerous as they accumulate in the body.

Extensive research into the true value of vitamins is growing daily, and the roles and inter-relationships of these essential nutrients is now understood to prevent a whole range of clinical deficiency symptoms. The most common general symptoms of vitamin deficiencies are lack of energy, constant infections, and retarded physical and mental development in children. Vitamins are essential to our health, development and well-being and the further detailed study of their use is essential to every therapist.

Minerals

Minerals are the *inorganic elements* that remain when living tissue of either plant or animal extraction is either compressed or burned. Minerals have many functions within the body and are considered to be essential when:

- a dietary shortage creates specific deficiency symptoms which normalise when the mineral is reintroduced at correct levels

- the addition of minerals to refined foods improves health
- it is seen to be a necessary co-factor in the operation and regulation of tissues, fluids, or enzymes, or as an important adjunct to the operation of other essential nutrients.

Minerals have three main functions:

- as the main constituents of bones and teeth – these include *calcium*, *magnesium* and *phosphorus*
- as soluble salts which control the composition of body fluids and cells – these include *sodium* and *chlorine* in the fluids (outside the cells) in blood and lymph, and *potassium*, *magnesium* and *phosphorus* (inside the cells)
- as essential co-factors in the production and use of many enzymes and proteins within the body (*iron*, *phosphorus* and many *trace elements*).

The body's concentration of minerals is maintained by absorption through the digestive system and excretion occurs through the kidneys, bile or intestinal secretions of various kinds. A dietary deficiency of either a mineral or a trace element can lead to a whole range of devastating deficiency diseases or conditions. It must however be remembered that excessive intake of some minerals and trace elements such as *cobalt*, *selenium*, *zinc* and *iron* can produce serious toxicity, so the body maintains its mineral balance within very narrow constraints. Like vitamins, minerals are worthy of further study as they are crucial to normal development and the maintenance of good health.

Sports therapy and the role of nutrition

Good nutrition is essential for all those who participate in sport, for no matter which sport or exercise we perform, we can improve our performance and capitalise on our training by changing our diet. How we store and use energy, the role of carbohydrates, fats and proteins in sport; and the way in which we can maximise the efficiency of vitamin and mineral absorption while training, are all part of the science of *Sports Nutrition*. This subject is too complex to cover here, but is covered in detail in the relevant ITEC courses.

It is essential that all therapists understand the complex subject of nutrition because it provides the very foundation of our development and our continuing health.

24 Physical Fitness and Aerobic Exercise

CONTRIBUTED BY SEAN BLAKE

The goal of every fitness instructor should be to help each of his or her clients to develop a balanced exercise programme that fits the specific needs, goals, lifestyle and limitations of each client. To accomplish this the instructor must first have a knowledge of the components of physical fitness, and the client's present level of fitness. This is covered in the first part of this chapter. Aerobic exercise is covered in the second part.

The components of physical fitness

The components of physical fitness are:

- health-related
- performance-related.

The health-related components

The health-related components of physical fitness are:

- *cardio-respiratory fitness* – the ability of the heart, blood vessels, blood and respiratory system to supply the working muscles with oxygen and nutrients. The working muscles especially require oxygen in order to function. A fit person can persist in physical activity for long periods of time without undue stress

- *muscular strength* – the ability to exert an external force or to lift a heavy object at least once

- *muscular endurance* – the ability to exert an external force or to lift a heavy object several times or to perform an exercise over a long period of time without the muscles becoming fatigued

- *body composition* – the quantification of the various components of the body, especially fat and muscle. A fit person has a relative low percentage of body fat

- *flexibility* – the ability of a joint (*articulation*) to move through its full range of motion.

The performance-related components

The performance-related components of physical fitness are:

- *speed* – the ability to perform a movement in a short period of time, for example sprinting
- *power* – the ability to transfer energy into force at a fast rate, for example throwing a javelin
- *agility* – the ability to change rapidly and accurately the position of one's body and to control the movement of the whole body, for example a gymnast
- *reaction time* – the time elapsed between simulation and the beginning of that simulation, for example a boxer deflecting a punch while delivering a blow at the same split second
- *co-ordination* – the ability to use the senses, with the body parts, to perform motor tasks smoothly and accurately, for example juggling.

It is impossible to design one or even several sample exercise programmes and expect them to meet the needs of every client you will encounter. But instructors are expected to use their knowledge and experience to develop a safe, effective, and enjoyable programme for each client.

Fitness evaluation

Every apparently healthy adult client is capable of achieving a level of fitness commensurate with his or her age and health. The instructor is responsible for assessing the client's current fitness status through health screening and fitness evaluation, clarifying measurable and realistic goals, and developing a programme that will help the client to accomplish those goals. A sound testing and evaluation package provides valuable information for both the instructor and the client. Additionally, it complements the instructor's exercise leadership skills, adds to the instructor's professional image, and is an additional revenue generating service which an instructor can provide.

The specific tests administered in an assessment will vary from individual to individual. A comprehensive assessment measures the following four components:

- cardio-respiratory efficiency
- muscular strength and endurance
- muscle and joint flexibility
- body composition.

The testing and evaluation process offers an opportunity to gather information related to the client's current level of physical fitness. Its purpose may be any of the following:

- to identify areas of health/injury risk and possible referral to the appropriate health professional
- to aid in the development of an exercise programme
- to establish goals and provide motivation
- to evaluate progress.

It is important to note that while many individuals look forward to their fitness testing and evaluation, some individuals may feel very uncomfortable with the process. Some individuals may be embarrassed with their present physical condition and a fitness evaluation may be counterproductive to the success of an exercise programme.

Health screening
The minimum evaluation an instructor should require is the completion of an *Exercise History and Health Screening Form* (see below). The screening form must be completed in order to determine the necessity of a physician's clearance and/or physician-supervised exercise testing.

The health history of a client is an instructor's primary tool for setting up a safe and effective exercise programme.

Health Screening Form

Name.. Date......................................

Physician's name...

Physician's telephone no...

Person to contact in case of emergency

Name........................... Relationship................. Telephone no......................

	Yes	No
Does you physician know that you are participating in this exercise programme?	☐	☐

Do you have, or have you had in the past:

		Yes	No
1	A history of heart problems, chest pain or stroke?	☐	☐
2	Increased blood pressure?	☐	☐
3	Any chronic illness or condition?	☐	☐
4	Difficulty with physical fitness?	☐	☐
5	Advice from your physician not to exercise?	☐	☐
6	Recent surgery (last 12 months)?	☐	☐
7	Pregnancy (now or within last 3 months)?	☐	☐
8	A history of breathing or lung problem?	☐	☐
9	Muscle, joint or back disorder, or any previous injury still affecting you?	☐	☐
10	Diabetes or thyroid condition?	☐	☐
11	Increased blood cholesterol?	☐	☐
12	history of heart problems in immediate family?	☐	☐
13	Hernia, or any condition that may be aggravated by lifting weights?	☐	☐
14	Cigarette smoking habit?	☐	☐
15	Obesity (more than 23% over ideal body weight)?	☐	☐

Comments...
....
....
....

Individuals who answer 'yes' to any of the questions 1–15 on the Health Screening Form above may be at increased risk of injury during exercise. These individuals should obtain a physician's release before starting an exercise programme. In addition, men over 40 years of age, women over 45 years of age, and any client with a medical condition the fitness instructor is not equipped to handle should obtain clearance from a physician.

The physician's release serves several purposes:

- It minimizes the individual's risk of injury.
- It reduces the instructor's liability.
- It enables the physician to direct modifications in the exercise programme.

Written consent   Everyone who is to be tested should read and sign an informed consent before being tested. This consent should explain the purpose and process of the testing, including a statement of the potential for discomfort, pain associated with the implementation of testing. It is the legal responsibility of the instructor to inform the person to be tested of even the most unlikely occurrences that could take place during a procedure. In the event of an incident, proper written emergency procedures and consents may help to protect the instructor or exercise facility, as long as the procedures were properly administered.

Fitness Testing

The fitness assessment is divided into two sections:

- *passive tests*
- *active tests*.

Passive tests   Passive tests involve:

- body weight check
- blood pressure reading
- resting heart rate measurement
- body composition measurements.

Body weight check

The client is asked to stand on a weighing scales while the instructor records the reading of the scales. Take note if the client has footwear on, so that this can be accounted for in the subsequent evaluation. It is recommended that the client is weighed without footwear.

Blood pressure reading

Blood pressure is measured with a *sphygmomanometer* and *stethoscope*. The sphygmomanometer consists of a rubber bladder enclosed in a nylon cuff and connected to an inflating bulb and manometer from which the pressure is read. It is important that the nylon cuff is placed correctly around the arm just above the elbow. The rubber tubing which extends from the cuff should be directly over the brachial artery on the inner portion of the elbow. The elbow should be slightly bent, the arm resting comfortably on a table or the arm of a chair. The stethoscope should come in contact with only the arm and should not touch any part of the cuff or tubing at the test site.

While listening carefully through the stethoscope, pump the cuff. The pulse should be heard then disappear as the cuff is pumped to approximately 20–30 mmHg above the point at which the sound disappeared. Release the pressure so that the pressure will fall about 2–3 mmHg/second. As the pressure falls, the sounds can be heard in four and sometimes five distinct phases, called *Korotkoff sounds*. The first sound heard is the first phase and represents the *systolic pressure* reading and should be noted. As the mercury continues to fall, this sound will change in quality to a louder, more sharp tapping representing the second and third phases which are of no particular significance. At rest, the fourth and fifth phases usually coincide and involve the disappearance of sound, which is the *diastolic pressure* reading and should be noted.

Note If a blood pressure measure needs to be repeated on the same arm, 30–60 seconds should be allowed for normal circulation to return. Results should be recorded for comparison with subsequent measurements. If there is significant discrepancy with readings from arm to arm, the client should be referred to his or her personal physician for medical evaluation, for such discrepancy may represent a significant circulatory problem.

Resting heart rate

The resting heart rate is usually measured *indirectly* by placing the fingertips on a pulse site (*palpation*), or *directly* by listening through a stethoscope (*auscultation*). The resting heart rate is most accurately measured just as the client gets out of bed in the morning.

Body composition

This refers to the quality or make up of *total body mass*. Total body mass can be divided into *lean body mass* and *fat mass*. Lean body mass is composed of bone, muscle, and organs. Fat body mass is composed of adipose tissue. The assessment of body composition determines the relative percentage of lean body mass and fat mass. The three most common methods of assessing body composition are:

- *Hydrostatic weighing* Also known as underwater weighing, this is considered the 'gold standard' of body composition assessment. The test involves suspending the subject, seated in a chair attached to a scale, in a tank of water. Body density is calculated from the relationship of normal body weight to underwater weight. From the body density, the percentage of body fat is calculated.

- *Bioelectrical impedance* The measurement of bioelectrical impedance is an increasingly popular method for determining body composition. It is based on the principle that the conductivity of an electrical impulse is greater through lean tissue that through fatty tissue. Pairs of electrodes, through which an imperceptible electrical current is passed, are placed on the hand and foot. The analyser, essentially an ohmmeter and a computer, measures the body's resistance to electrical flow in ohms, and from that computes body density and percentage body fat. The subject should be well hydrated and not have exercised in the previous six hours or consumed alcohol in the previous 12 hours. Assessing body composition via bioelectrical impedance is both fast, easy, and requires minimal technical training.

- *Skinfold measurements* Measurements of skinfold provides a relatively inexpensive way to assess body composition. The results are both valid and reliable if the measurements are taken properly. The standard error of the method is 3.5 per cent or more fat, depending on the equation applied. This is compared to a 2.7 per cent error for a hydrostatically determined measurement. The method, based on the notion that approximately 50 per cent of total body fat is under the skin, involves measuring the thickness of the skinfold sites. These measurements are summed and applied to one of many equations available. Calipers specifically designed for skinfold measurement are the only equipment needed for this method of body fat assessment. The procedure for measuring skinfolds is as follows:

1 Identify the anatomical location of the skinfold. All measurements are taken on the right side of the body.

2 Grasp the skinfold firmly with the thumb and index finger of the left hand.

3 Place the calipers in the correct position, one quarter inch from the thumb and forefinger.

4 Read the measurement to the nearest 0.5 millimetre, one or two seconds after the trigger has been released.

5 A minimum of two measurements should be taken on each site.

Active tests Active testing requires the client to perform tasks which will place him or her under physical stress. It is very important that the instructor observes the client for distress and acts accordingly.

The active tests are divided into four areas:

- muscular strength
- muscular endurance
- flexibility
- cardio-respiratory fitness.

Testing muscular strength and endurance

Adequate muscular strength and endurance are necessary for both optimal health and optimal athletic performance. From a health perspective, adequate strength and endurance facilitate participation in activities of daily living without injury or undue fatigue, and also enhance life at an optimal level of human function.

Dynamometer grip strength test   The dynamometer may be used to test several groups of muscles. In this evaluation it is used to test the strength of the client's grip strength.

1   Adjust the dynamometer to fit the size of the client's hand by turning the easily adjustable screw located at the top.

2   The client stands straight, knees slightly soft, arms by his or her side.

3   The client grips and squeezes the handle on the dynamometer as hard as he or she can.

4   Read the score on the dynamometer dial and record the score.

5   Do the test twice on each hand and take the average reading of the four readings.

Sit-up test (abdominals)   The equipment requirements for a sit-up test are a stopwatch and an exercise mat.

1   Ask the client to lie face up with knees bent at right angles and heels about 15–18 inches from the buttocks, hands cupping the ears.

2   Hold the client's ankles firmly to keep the feet in contact with the floor.

3   Count the number of sit-ups performed in one minute. The client's shoulders should touch the floor to complete each sit-up.

Note: In order to avoid neck injury, the client should be warned not to pull on the neck and head and to keep the buttocks on the mat.

Press-up test (triceps, anterior deltoids, pectoralis major)   Press-up position for men: the hands and toes only touching the floor. Press-up position for women: use modified bent-knee position.

1   The client should assume the appropriate starting position with the hands about a shoulder width apart.

2   Ensure that the exercises are performed correctly.

3   Count the number of press-ups performed in one minute.

Testing flexibility

Flexibility is defined as the range of motion of a given joint. Flexibility affects both health and fitness, inflexibility increases risk of joint and muscle injury. The most frequent example is lower back inflexibility, which relates to low back pain and injury.

Sit and reach (trunk flexion)

1   Place a yard stick on the floor, place a piece of tape 12 inches long at right angles to the stick at the 15 inch mark on the stick.

2   Ask the client to sit on the floor, removing his or her shoes.

3   The client sits with the stick between the legs, with the zero mark towards the body.

4   The feet should be 12 inches apart and the heels aligned with the tape at the 15 inch mark on the yard stick.

5   With one hand on the other, and with the fingers aligned, the client exhales and slowly leans forward.

6   Fingers in contact with the yardstick, the client reaches as far as possible. Record the distance reached.

Note: A small warm-up is advisable before performing this test in order to prevent injury to the lower back. The client should keep the knees soft while performing this test.

Shoulder flexibility   Swimming, tennis and throwing sports all require flexibility in the shoulder for good performance and avoidance of injury. The purpose of the test of shoulder flexibility is to measure the multi-rotational components of the shoulder joints.

1   The client should place the right hand on the right shoulder, gradually moving down the back, bending the left arm, sliding the left hand behind and up the back.

2   The client must now try to bring both hands together until they touch, or as close as possible.

3   Measure the amount of flexibility in the shoulders by the distance covered by the hands. It will be a plus or minus reading.

4   Repeat the test procedure for the opposite shoulder.

Testing cardio-respiratory fitness (sub-maximal)

Step test   This test involves the delivery of a measured aerobic stimulus controlled by stepping to a standardised cadence. It requires less cost, and can be used in mass testing situations.

Equipment needed:

- a 12-inch step
- a metronome for accurate pacing (96 bpm)
- a stopwatch.

1   Set the metronome to 96 bpm (24 cycles per minute).

2   The client starts stepping to a four-beat cycle – up, up, down, down.

3   Both feet must make contact with the top of the step at the upper portion of the cycle, and make contact with the floor on the down position.

4   Stepping will last for three minutes.

5   Immediately after the stepping, the client should sit for a one-minute pulse count. The one-minute post-exercise heartrate is used to score the test.

Note: Start the timing of the three minutes when the subject starts stepping. Stop the exercise if the client is showing distress.

The Rockport walk test (1 mile)   This is routinely used to assess cardiovascular fitness. The test involves a timed one-mile walk/run on a smooth and level surface (preferably a quarter of a mile running track). The only equipment needed is a stopwatch.

An advantage of this test over the lab tests is that it evaluates *performance*, whereas the lab tests measure *parameters* (e.g. estimated CO_2, workload, or heartrate) that give a very good indication of how well an individual will perform during an aerobic activity. The limitations to the test lie in the fact that pacing ability and body fat weight may adversely affect performance.

1 Begin with a warm-up.

2 Explain to the client that the test requires maximum effort. Make it clear that if at any time the client feels distress, he or she may pull out.

3 Immediately upon completion, take a ten-second pulse count and record the result.

4 The client should cool down for five minutes once the test is completed.

Aerobic exercise

Aerobic exercise to music was virtually unknown in the 1970s. However, in recent years it has become one of the most popular forms of exercise. The term aerobic means 'with oxygen' or 'in the presence of oxygen', but it has become synonymous in the public mind with exercise to music, of which there are many different types:

- aerobic dance
- step aerobics
- aqua aerobics
- circuit aerobics

with the list growing annually. The increase in interest is well-deserved. A good aerobics programme can improve aspects of aerobic conditioning, flexibility, strength and agility as well as provide a safe and sociable form of exercise.

The structure of an aerobics class

An aerobics class should be similar in structure to other aerobic fitness programmes. There should be four phases:

- *warm-up phase* – dynamic movement, mobility movement, pre-stretch
- *aerobic phase* – non/low/high impact/intensity movement
- *conditioning phase* – muscular strength and endurance exercise
- *cool-down phase* – developmental stretching and relaxation.

Each phase should have a pulse-check included. The importance of pulse-taking cannot be over-emphasised – it is an indicator of how well an individual is coping with the exercise. If the pulse rate is monitored throughout the workout, the instructor can see that the benefit for each individual is achieved.

Each individual should be taught how to take his or her own pulse. Show them the two areas most commonly used:

- the wrist (radial artery)
- the neck (carotid artery).

If a person cannot find his or her own pulse, you should help them. The pulse is taken for 6 seconds and multiplied by 10 in order to get the 60-second count.

The four pulse-checks which should be carried out are:

- at the start of the class
- before the pre-stretch
- at the end of the aerobic phase
- at the end of the class.

The warm-up phase

The warm-up phase includes:

- *dynamic movement* – a general warm-up achieved by using the major muscle groups in a controlled, brisk, rhythmical activity
- *mobility movement* – achieved in conjunction with the warm-up movements by ensuring all the joints (articulations) are taken through a wide range of movement
- *pre-stretch* (static stretching) – specific static stretching is recommended. The sites commonly needing attention for the class are the calf, hamstrings, quadricep, lower back and adductors.

The purpose of the warm-up phase is to:

- to prepare the body for exercise
- reduce the risk of injury
- improve the performance in physical activity.

These are guidelines for a successful warm-up:

- Simple movements – don't make people feel awkward.
- It should last at least ten minutes depending on conditions, i.e. hot weather or cool weather.
- The pulse should rise up to 100–110 (approx.).
- All movements should be smooth and controlled.
- Participants should break into a light sweat.
- Specific muscles and joints should be put through their actions.
- Comfort zone: participants should feel part of the class and not feel excluded. The class should be advertised to suit either beginners, intermediate, and/or intermediate to advanced abilities.

The *physiological benefits of the warm-up* are:

- increased delivery of oxygen to the working muscles
- raised temperature of extremities to that of the core and increased circulation
- more forceful and rapid muscle contraction when warm
- more rapid travel of nerve impulses, increased sensitivity of the nerve, improved co-ordination, quicker reflexes
- improved cardiovascular response to sudden strenuous exercise
- improved flexibility of muscles when warm – cold muscles are less elastic and therefore may be more susceptible to damage. Flexibility of tendons and ligaments is also affected by an increase in temperature.

Note: Warm-up will help to eliminate any stiffness and tension in the muscle, tendons and joints. Flexibility will increase, thus helping the body to absorb stress and cope more efficiently.

The aerobic phase

The immediate aim of the aerobic phase is to provide a controlled duration of exercise at the right level and for the right length of time to induce the cardio-respiration training effect. For an individual to get the most benefit from the aerobics class, he or she must be working (exercising) at the right intensity for their present fitness level. This can be achieved by:

- establishing his or her *resting heartrate*, and then
- using the *Karvonen Formula* to calculate the *training heartrate*:

Method			*Example*		
220			220		
−	Minus the age		−	30	Minus age
=	Max. *heart rate*		=	190	Max. *heart rate*
−	Minus the resting heartrate		−	70	Resting heartrate
=	Heartrate reserve		=	120	Heartrate reserve
×	0.6 (60%) of max. heartrate		×	0.6	(60%) of max. heartrate
=			=	72.0	
+	Resting heartrate		+	70	Resting heartrate
=	*Training heartrate*		=	142	*Training heartrate*

The *training heartrate* (THR) should be 60–80 per cent of the *maximum heartrate* (MHR). The lower threshold has now been calculated (142 bpm) and equals 60 per cent of the maximum heart rate. For the individual to receive any benefit from the exercise class, he or she must increase the heartrate to *at least* 142 bpm. The exact same formula would be used to get the higher threshold, by multiplying the heart rate reserve by 0.8 (80 per cent) of the maximum heart rate. The goal of the individual is to work (exercise) between the two thresholds to achieve the training effect.

The aerobic energy system   The main supply of fuel to the aerobic system is in the form of carbohydrates (glucose) and fat (fatty acids), which are converted into adenosine triphosphate (ATP). ATP is the body's energy source, just as petrol is the energy source in a car. While there is some ATP stored in the muscle cell, the supply is limited. Therefore, muscle cells must produce more ATP in order to continue working. Most cells, including muscle cells, contain structures called *mitochondria*. The mitochondria are the sites of aerobic energy (ATP) production. The greater the number of mitochondria in a cell, the greater the aerobic energy production capability of that cell.

Characteristics of aerobic exercise

- Rhythmic exercise at a steady sustained pace over an extended period: 20–45 minutes.
- Exercises that involve large muscle groups: quadriceps/hamstrings/calves.

- Exercise that requires large amounts of blood to be transported to the tissue via the circulatory system.
- The body can cope with the demands being made for full duration.

Types of aerobic exercise include: aerobic dance, step aerobics, aqua aerobics, walking, cycling.

Intensity of aerobic exercise   The physiological stress on the body during exercise indicates how hard the body should be working to achieve a training effect.

The aerobic phase should always begin with low *impact* (low intensity) exercise and gradually increase to medium impact and to high impact exercise and tapering off at low impact:

LOW   →   MEDIUM   →   HIGH   →   MEDIUM   →   LOW.

- *Low impact* – one foot is in contact with the floor at all times.
- *Medium impact* – a balance of low/high impact, i.e. a light skip with a hop.
- *High impact* – both feet leave the ground at the same time, i.e. jumping jacks/skipping.

Note: There should be no more than 24 continuous high impact moves at any one time.

The increases *intensity* in an aerobic phase is achieved by:

- bigger leg movements
- bigger arm movements, with adequate rest due to fatigue
- increased speed/directional changes.

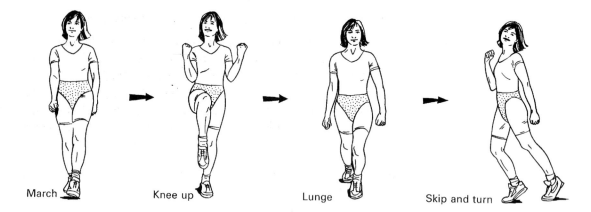

March   Knee up   Lunge   Skip and turn

EXAMPLES OF AN
AEROBIC SEQUENCE

Therefore, there is a difference between high impact and higher intensity – both can be performed separately or together. For example, a jumping jack is a high-impact move which can be performed with no arm movements. However, if the arms are raised overhead while performing the jumping jacks, the result will be *high impact/high intensity*.

- *Low intensity* – arms *below the heart* as in biceps curl exercise.
- *High intensity* – arms *above the heart* as in shoulder press exercise.

The conditioning phase

The conditioning phase is designed to promote muscular strength using exercises involving resistance through gravity, body weight, a partner and equipment such as hand weights and rubber bands. The aim is to:

- make all the muscles strong enough to support the skeletal structure
- maintain posture and body shape
- improve overall strength, so that the body can take part in an activity that involves continuous use of the muscles for normal day-to-day activities.

Standard exercises involved in the conditioning phase include:

- *for the upper body* – press ups (triceps/pectorals), shoulder press (deltoids/trapezius), upright row (trapezius)
- *for the mid section* – curl-ups (rectus abdominus), reverse curls (transversus abdominus), oblique twists (internal/external obliques), back extensions (erector spinae).
- *for the lower body* – hip extensions (glutus maximus and hamstrings), side leg raise (abductors), inner thigh raise (adductors), calf raise (gastrocnemius).

Note: It is important that the correct form is adhered to when performing the above exercises. The class will copy (mirror) the instructor's posture and movements, so the instructor should beware of his or her own body positioning.

The strength exercises performed are of the following types:

- *isotonic* – a muscular contraction in which the muscle exerts a constant tension, for example press-up exercise, curl up 'abdominal' exercise or biceps curl with resistance using weights.
- *isometric* (*static*) – a muscular contraction where no change in the length of the muscle takes place, for example by performing a press-up exercise and holding that position without moving, or performing a leg raise and holding the leg in that position.

Note: All isometric exercises should only be held for the count of six to eight seconds.

Training principles for the conditioning phase are:

- Exercises for all major muscle groups should be included, particularly those not worked during the aerobic phase.
- Avoid creating local fatigue, shift work from muscle group to muscle group, ensuring smooth transitions.
- High repetition and low resistance are required for muscular endurance.
- Low repetition and high resistance are required for muscular strength.

211

The challenge in the conditioning phase is to strike a balance between the four principles. This can be achieved by giving careful consideration to the implementation of progression.

The cool-down phase

As with the warm-up, a cool-down period is a vital component of any exercise session. It involves a gradual decrease in the intensity of the exercise until the body's physiological functions return to the resting state. A successful cool-down helps the muscles of the body return blood to the heart so that it does not pool in the muscles.

It is important to emphasise the importance of the cool-down in relation to flexibility and mobility of the joints, and the suppleness of the muscles. The cool-down exercises should be slow, smooth and sustained. Each exercise (stretch) should be held for 30 seconds to the point of tension, but not pain. Breathing should be slow and regular to give a sense of complete relaxation and refreshment. Relaxation should be the aim to bring about the sensation of a body and mind completely free of tension.

Some important exercise considerations

It is important to consider the following points:

- Injured clients should not take part in high-impact aerobics.
- Suitable clothing and footwear must be worn.
- Extra care should be taken with overweight, unfit, elderly, pregnant or injured clients.
- The instructor must be able to adapt all high moves to low-impact moves when needed.
- Aerobic exercise should be progressive, enjoyable, and non-competitive.
- Instructors should observe clients for signs of distress during the activity.
- Correct flooring, i.e. wooden sprung flooring, should be used at all times. If not, the exercises must be modified to suit the space available.
- Avoid joint and muscle overuse/overload.
- The instructor should alter the duration and intensity of the aerobic activity to suit a particular class: elderly, beginner, intermediate or advanced.

Benefits of aerobic exercise

The long-term health benefits of aerobic exercise are:

- improved cardiac efficiency, improved stroke volume (that is, quantity of blood pumped per heart beat)
- a lower resting heartrate
- favourable changes in body composition, increase in lean body mass (muscle mass)
- improved quality of life and reduced risk of hypokinetic/chronic diseases.

Exercise cueing

Effective exercise cueing distinguishes the good instructor from the average instructor. This is because the class participants always follow the instructor's first movement, and if it is wrong, the fluency of the class is lost and the instructor loses credibility. It is important, then, that the instructor always uses good cueing techniques when changing from one exercise to another.

Cues may be defined as:

- *Verbal*:
    - direction and placement – (voice projection) tell where to go
    - countdown/timing – how many to go/where to change
    - technique/quality – signal change in intensity, pace and rhythm.
- *Non-verbal*:
    - facial expression – smile/eye contact, etc.
    - music – contains built-in cues that are in rhythm, phrasing and lyric composition
    - signs or symbols – hand signals or cards, etc.
    - exercise selection and progression – logical and simple steps make cueing easier
    - props/whistles, cue cards/circuit cards.

Music and the exercise class

Music is an important element in an aerobic class. It:

- motivates
- relieves boredom and offers variety
- aids correct timing and co-ordination
- encourages creativity and enjoyment
- helps the instructor.

Selecting music

- *for the warm-up phase* (125 bpm to 135 bpm) choose lively, familiar music with a steady tempo (not too fast).
- *for the aerobic phase* (130 bpm to 165 bpm) choose lively, popular, motivational music with a regular beat. Change the music to suit high and low-impact exercises.
- *for the conditioning phase* (120 bpm to 125 bpm) choose music with a steady beat but not fast and with no change of tempo. It should be motivational.
- *for the cool-down phase* choose a slow, relaxing instrumental. No beat is necessary as it may encourage jerking.

Guidelines for organising aerobic classes

- Participants must fill out Health Screen Questionnaire.
- The class must include a warm-up.
- No one should be allowed onto the floor after the warm-up has started.

- Well-cushioned footwear is compulsory.
- Participants should be advised to exercise *before* eating rather than after eating.
- Participants should be encouraged to attend class on a regular basis.
- The instructor should be positioned in such a way that he or she can view the entire class.
- The class should be specific to the level of fitness of the participants.
- The instructor should have an *emergency plan* in case of an accident:
  - have a knowledge of first aid and/or CPR
  - carry a first aid kit
  - know where the nearest telephone is
  - have an emergency contact number.
- The instructor should have a knowledge of some of the contra-indications to aerobic exercises, and use this knowledge with skill and commonsense when teaching aerobic exercise. Aerobic exercise is contra-indicated by:
  - incorrect posture, which can lead to injury – must be corrected immediately
  - exercise involving deep knee bends – must be corrected immediately, if observed
  - hyperextension – must be corrected immediately, if observed
  - too much overload/intensity, which will cause acute and/or chronic injuries
  - bouncing on toes, which will cause shin splints/bone fractures
  - incorrect footwear, giving little protection, which can cause injury to the ankle, leg, hip and spine
  - overcrowding, which may cause injury (It is illegal to take an overcrowded class.)
  - poor ventilation – lack of oxygen may cause injury and even death
  - ballistic-type stretching, which will cause injury to muscles/tendons
  - participants on medication – if in doubt, instructor should advise against participation
  - obesity (overweight by 23 per cent) – physician's clearance recommended.
  - Anorexia nervosa (obsessive desire to lose weight by refusing to eat) – if known, it is essential to get a physician's written and verbal clearance before accepting the client into the class.

It is important that an instructor keeps up-to-date with changes in the fitness field. This can be done by up-dating his or her qualifications, reading health and fitness articles, and by attending health and fitness workshops and seminars.

25 Resistance Training and Gym Instruction

CONTRIBUTED BY SEAN BLAKE

Resistance, strength and weight-training have become a popular form of recreation as well as a way of conditioning athletes. This type of exercise requires the body's musculature to move (or attempt to move) against an opposing force presented by various types of equipment. We use the term *resistance training* to describe this type of exercise, rather than 'weight-training', which really refers to a performance characteristic of muscle function and may be defined as the maximal force a muscle or muscle group can generate at a specified velocity. The most commonly used forms of resistance exercise are free weights and weight machines.

Demonstrations of strength have captured the interest and imagination of people as far back as ancient times. Resistance training is said to have begun when the Greek god Milo carried a calf on his shoulders daily until it became a bull.

Many colleges and professional sports teams today have full-time strength and conditioning instructors. Health clubs are filled with resistance-training enthusiasts. Colleges and universities are offering resistance-training courses to thousands of students. People who do resistance training on a regular basis do so for one or more of the following reasons:

- to improve health status
- to reproportion or sculpture their bodies for appearance's sake
- for competition purpose (Olympic-style weight-lifting, power-lifting), body building and athletic performance.

There is little doubt that resistance-training has gained universal acceptance as an expedient method for accomplishing these outcomes. The dark ages for resistance training, marked by myths, has given way to scientific evidence encouraging its use, allied with an enlightened understanding of its benefits.

215

Strength benefits of resistance training

Strength training is the process of exercising with progressively heavier resistance for the purpose of strengthening the musculoskeletal system. Physiologically the positive adaptation which results from regular training includes:

- increased muscle fibre size
- increased muscle contractile strength
- increased tendon tensile strength
- increased ligament tensile strength
- increased bone tensile strength.

These beneficial changes in the musculoskeletal tissue have a profound influence on:

- *physical capacity*   This may be defined as a person's ability to perform work or exercise. Muscles utilise energy to produce movement power, functioning as the engines of our bodies. Specifically, strength training increases the size and strength of our muscle fibres, resulting in a greater physical capacity to perform work.
- *physical appearance*   Our skeletal muscles have a lot to do with our overall physique. Consequently, strength training can play a major role in enhancing our body composition and physical appearance.
- *metabolic function*   Muscle is very active tissue with high energy requirements for maintenance and rebuilding processes. Even as we sleep, our skeletal muscles are responsible for over 25 per cent of our calorie use. An increase in muscle tissue causes a corresponding increase in our metabolic rate, and a decrease in muscle tissue causes a corresponding decrease in our metabolic rate.
- *injury risk*   In addition to being the engines of the body, our muscles also serve as shock absorbers and balancing agents. Strong muscles helps dissipate the repetitive landing forces experienced in weight-bearing activities such as running and aerobic dance. Balanced muscle development reduces the risk of over-use injuries which result when one muscle group is much stronger than its opposing muscle group.

Muscle action

It is important for a gym instructor to have a sound knowledge of anatomy and physiology, and to understand the actions of specific muscles in relation to the stress placed upon them when performing an exercise. The three types of muscle actions are:

- *dynamic concentric (positive) contraction*, which occurs when the muscle contracts and shortens and movement takes place. For example, a dynamic contraction of the thigh contracts and the knee joint extends.
- *dynamic eccentric (negative) contraction*, which occurs when the muscle contracts and lengthens and the movement takes place. For example, lowering a weight from the extended knee position is a dynamic eccentric contraction of the quadriceps.

216

- *isometric (static) contraction*, where the muscle contracts, but no movement occurs, for example, when a lifter attempts to perform a leg press or with a resistance that he or she cannot lift.

Joint action

An articulation, or joint, is the point of connection between bones, or bones and cartilage. The stability and integrity of all the joints are maintained by ligaments, which are dense fibrous strands of connective tissue that link the bony segments together. Some joints permit a large range of motion in several directions, while other joints permit virtually no motion at all.

The various joints in the body can be classified into two general categories according to:

- the structure of the joint
- the type of movement allowed by the joint.

If the resistance training is performed by using incorrect lifting techniques or using too much overload, it will undoubtedly place one or more articulations at risk. It is important that the instructor should have a thorough knowledge and understanding of the workings of the joints in relation to their functions. If resistance training is performed correctly, as in the use of free weights where the individual has to balance the resistance rather than be guided by machinery, the controlling action is an aid in the development of the joint.

Resistance training

There are four categories of resistance training:

- *dynamic constant (isotonic) resistance training*
- *dynamic variable (isotonic) resistance training*
- *isokinetic resistance training*
- *isometric resistance training*

Dynamic constant resistance training

This is defined as a 'muscular contraction in which the muscle exerts a constant tension'. The execution of free-weight exercise and exercises on various weight-training machines, though usually considered isotonic are not by nature isotonic. The tension exerted by a muscle in the performance of such exercises is not constant, but varies with the mechanical advantage of the joint involved in the movement. A more workable definition of isotonic is 'a resistance training exercise where the external resistance or weight does not vary'. Because there is confusion concerning the term isotonic, most people have adopted the term *dynamic constant resistance training*.

The advantages of dynamic constant resistance exercise include low cost of equipment, similarity to most work and exercise activities, variety of training movement, tangible evidence of improvement and easy accessibility.

217

The disadvantages include the inability to train through a full range of motion in many exercises, and inconsistent matching of resistive forces and muscular forces throughout the exercise movement.

Dynamic variable resistance training

This training requires equipment similar to that of dynamic constant resistance training in that the amount of resistive force encountered determines the amount of muscle force applied. However, it is different in that the resistive force changes throughout the exercise movement. Variable resistance equipment operates through a lever arm, cam or pulley arrangement. Its purpose is to alter the resistance throughout the range of motion of an exercise in an attempt to match the increase and decreases in exercise. By increasing and decreasing the resistance to match the strength curve of the exercise, the muscle is forced to contract maximally throughout the range of motion resulting in maximum gains in strength.

The advantages of dynamic variable resistance exercise include the ability to train through a full range of joint motion on most exercises, reasonably consistent matching of resistive forces and muscular forces throughout the exercise movement, and in most cases tangible evidence of improvement.

The disadvantage include equipment expense, limited number of training movements and lack of accessibility.

Isokinetic resistance training

Isokinetic refers to a muscular contraction performed at a constant angular limb velocity. Unlike other types of resistance training, there is no set resistance to meet, but rather the velocity of movement is controlled. That is, the amount of muscle force applied determines the amount of resistance encountered. More muscle force produces more resistive force, and vice versa. Isokinetic machines normally have an electrically braked, mechanically braked or hydraulic system that attempts to make the velocity of the movement constant. Due to the need for acceleration and deceleration during the movement, a true isokinetic contraction may only occur in approximately the middle third of the movement. Isokinetic machines are popular because they cause less muscular soreness than other forms of resistance training, at least during the initial training sessions.

Various isokinetic machines allow for no eccentric phase (muscle lengthening) of muscle contraction as one gets when lowering a weight. This lack of an eccentric contraction is in part responsible for the reduced muscle soreness. It is important to note that eccentric strength is used in many athletic events and daily living activities. Simply walking down steps involves eccentric contractions of the quadriceps. In addition, eccentric contractions may be a vital part of the stimulus to promote strength gains and muscle growth.

The advantages of isokinetic exercise include accommodating resistance forces, speed regulation and detailed performance feedback.

The disadvantages include cost of equipment, force regulation, need for training motivation and lack of accessibility.

Isometric resistance training

This refers to a muscular contraction where no change in the length of the muscle takes place. This type of resistance training is normally performed against an immovable object such as a wall, a weight machine or barbell loaded beyond the maximal concentric of the individual. Isometric exercises can also be performed by having a weak muscle group contract against a strong muscle group. For example, trying to bend the right elbow and resisting the movement by pushing down on the right hand with the left hand for a maximum of eight seconds. The right elbow flexors are weaker than the left elbow extensors, so the right biceps would be performing an isometric contraction. It is important to note that one should breathe normally while performing this type of exercise.

The advantages of isometric resistance training include little equipment needed, low cost, space efficiency, and time efficiency.

The disadvantages include increased blood pressure, increased strength only at specifically exercised positions in the movement range, lack of performance feedback.

Resistance training equipment

Free-weight exercises

The advantages of free-weight training are progressive resistance, wide variety of exercise, unlimited movement patterns, and the incorporation of assistance muscle groups for balance and stability.

The disadvantages are training time, exercise control, and injury risk.

All free-weight exercise should be performed through a full range of motion, with controlled movement speed and continuous breathing.

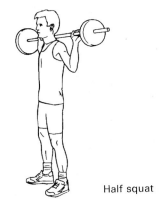
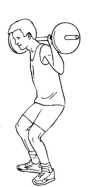
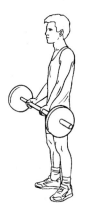
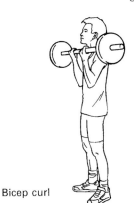

Half squat   Bicep curl

EXAMPLES OF FREE-WEIGHT EXERCISES

Machine exercises

The advantages of machine training are supportive structure, variable resistance, rotary movement. These features contribute to exercise safety and muscle isolation.

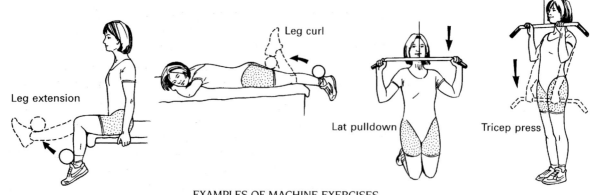

Leg extension

Leg curl

Lat pulldown

Tricep press

EXAMPLES OF MACHINE EXERCISES

The disadvantages are space consumption (depending on size of machine) and limited number of exercises stations on the machine.

Body weight exercise The advantages of body weight exercise are low cost (no equipment) and easy accessibility. The disadvantages are lack of progressive resistance and difficulty in targeting specific muscle groups.

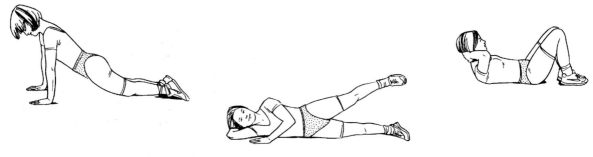

EXAMPLES OF FLOOR CONDITIONING EXERCISES

High-risk exercise equipment There are hundreds of strength training exercises and nearly the same amount of exercise equipment, each one is effective to some degree. However, many exercises commonly performed by body-builders and weightlifters pose a high risk of injury for average strength-training individuals. It is the role of the qualified gym/fitness instructor to match the exercise and equipment to an individual's needs, ensuring safety and effectiveness.

Compound and isolation exercise training

Having selected the right equipment, the next step is to select the most appropriate exercise. There are two types of exercise:

- *compound exercises*, which involve more than one major muscle or muscle group. Because of the large muscle mass involved, this type of exercise uses more energy and is therefore better for overall conditioning and weight loss programmes.

220

- *isolation exercises*, in which a specific muscle is isolated for the purpose of strengthening or enlarging that muscle. This type of exercise generally involves little overall energy use and is more specific to strength-training or body-building programmes.

A beginner would concentrate on compound movements, while the advanced person would use a mixture of compound/isolation exercises.

There are many compound and isolation exercises available. However, a selection of five of the best of each can give a variety of exercises, which in total or in some combination can be used in any resistance-training programme. The following are examples of both compound and isolation resistance exercise (note that they are not in a specific order). A person should consult with his or her instructor before commencing a resistance-training programme.

Examples of compound and isolation exercises:

- *compound* – benchpress, lat pulldown, press-up, squats, leg extension
- *isolation* – concentrated bicep curl, wrist curl, hammer curl, abdominal crunch.

Designing a resistance-training programme

Before designing a resistance training programme, it is important to perform a *needs analysis*, which involves simply determining the client's needs. The easiest way to conduct a needs analysis is for the client to answer a series of questions concerning his or her desired goals, then the instructor can determine specific goals for the resistance-training programme. Some common goals of resistance-training programmes are as follows:

- increased strength/power of specific muscle groups
- increased local muscular endurance of specific muscle groups
- increased motor performance, i.e. increased ability to run, jump, throw
- increased total body weight
- increased muscle hypertrophy
- decreased body fat.

It is possible to achieve all of these goals with a well-planned and well-balanced resistance training programme. However, the expected changes in these characteristics must be kept within reasonable limits, depending on the age of the client and his or her biological potential for change.

For a resistance-training programme to be safe and effective, the principles of training must be adhered to:

- *specificity*
- *overload*
- *progression*
- *recuperation*
- *reversibility*.

221

Specificity   Specificity of training implies that different forms of exercise produce different results. The type of exercise carried out is specific both to the muscle group being used and to the energy source involved. The instructor/trainer will need to decide which type of muscle resistance (e.g. isometric, isokinetic, isotonic resistance) should be used to achieve the most effective results. Specificity is a major tenet in resistance training. It assumes that muscles show the greatest evidence of strength increase in activities similar to the training exercise in terms of:

- the body around which movement occurs
- the joint range of motion
- the pattern of resistance throughout the range of motion
- the pattern of limb velocity throughout the range of motion
- whether the movement is concentric, eccentric, isometric.

Overload   Overload is the key concept in exercise programming. This implies that an individual must not exercise at a level above that which is comfortable. As fitness levels improve, so the training threshold can be raised. Think FITT:

- *frequency* – training sessions: How many times per day/week/month?
- *intensity*
  - heartrate (training threshold)
  - resistance/repetitions/sets
  - movement – fast or slow
- *time* – training time per session
- *type* – type of exercise: anaerobic or aerobic.

Progression   As an individual becomes more fit, a higher intensity of exercise is required to create an overload and therefore provide continued improvements. Progression can be through either increased intensity or duration of exercise sessions.

General guidelines

- Overall increases should not exceed 10 per cent each week.
- Progression is achieved by increasing any of the overload variables.

Recuperation   Rest is essential between training sessions to allow for adaptation. Muscles need to adapt to the stress of the exercise, thus preventing too much overload, which in turn will cause injury. Recuperation allows time for tissue recovery and fuel replacement.

Recuperation within a workout

- *Work: recovery ratio* A period of rest should be given between each exercise, e.g. circuit training.
- *Low/high intensity* The muscles should be worked continuously, but without causing fatigue by including low-intensity recovery.
- *Cool-down period* This allows for the muscles to return to a normal state, and is achieved by performing low-intensity exercise, stretching exercise and relaxation techniques.

Recuperation between workouts

- *Adaptation* With a period of rest and proper progression the muscles will adapt to the specific exercise/overload.

- *Tissue recovery and repair* This will only take place during the period of rest.

- *Fuel replacement* This is essential if the muscles are to continue working.

- *Relaxation/sleep* This allows time for the physiological and psychological recovery of body tissues.

Reversibility   Training effects are reversible in that if the training stops for a period of time due to injury, or if it is not often enough or intense enough, loss of benefits can quickly occur. This can be prevented by continuing training at a maintenance level after a high level of conditioning has been obtained. Factors which can affect the reversibility process:

- Length of layoff. If you do not use it (i.e. exercise), you will lose it. The longer the layoff, the more gains that will be lost.

- Fitness level will determine the speed at which any gains may be lost. The fitter the individual, the better their chance of retaining the gains made.

- The number of years of training. A conditioned body will retain all its gains for longer than an unconditioned body.

- Appropriate restart: It is important to *think safe*. An individual should start at his or her present level of fitness and not at the point at which he or she stopped.

Note: An individual should build on their fitness and not on their injuries.

The programme card or
training chart   The instructor should record in a programme card or training chart the number of sets, repetitions, and resistance for each exercise in a training session. This information is useful in several ways:

- It demonstrates the progress of each lifter in terms of resistance used and repetitions performed, information that can be motivational for the lifter.

- It helps the instructor to evaluate the success of the training programme and determine when the resistance should be increased for a particular exercise.

- It is a reminder of the order of the exercise to be performed, the resistance to be used, and number of repetitions to be performed during the training session.

Some training programmes allow the user to record total body weight prior to each training session. This is useful, especially if the individual is attempting to lose or gain weight. Training charts may also have a section for modifications/comments concerning the training session, such as whether the session seems easy or difficult.

223

| Name | Age |
| Week | Day | Weight | kg |

Exercise	¹ Weight	Reps	Sets	² Weight	Reps	Sets	³ Weight	Reps	Sets
Benchpress									
Leg extension									
Lat pulldown									
Leg curl									
Incline flye									
Squat									
Rhomboid row									
Deltoid raise									
Calf raise									
Abdominal curl									
Back extension									

Comments

Exercise modifications

EXAMPLE OF A
PROGRAMME CARD
(TRAINING CHART)

The training chart above can document three sets of exercise per training session per week. It allows the user to record total body weight prior to each training session and to note necessary equipment modifications.

Contra-indications to resistance training

Resistance training is contra-indicated by:

- incorrect instruction
- incorrect lifting technique
- intensity/overload too high
- spotter* inattentive
- the misuse or lack of collars on free weights
- failing to follow the resistance programme as set out by the instructor
- insufficient hygiene practice within the training facility.

Note: All equipment should be checked for faulty parts. Equipment should be cleaned on a daily basis.

* *Spotter*: A training partner (instructor or friend) who gives assistance to an unsuccessful lifting attempt, provides encouragement and feedback, and helps the exerciser to train in a safe and effective manner.

Guidelines for safe, effective resistance training

An instructor must completely understand safe exercise technique before attempting to teach an exercise to an individual, whether that person is a beginner or an advanced exerciser. Good spotting technique is vital for a safe resistance-training programme. The following is a spotter's checklist:

- Start with an adequate warm-up.
- Know proper exercise technique:
  - *Base* – the lifter must first be in the correct position
  - *Back* – correct posture will insure the lifter's lower back is safe
  - *Breathing* – checking that the lifter exhales on the exertion.
- The instructor must be strong enough to assist the lifter with the resistance that he or she is lifting.
- Know how many repetitions the lifter intends to do.
- Be attentive to the lifter at all times.
- Stop the exercise if it is performed incorrectly.
- Heavy resistance should not be used until lifting techniques are perfected.
- The exercise should involve opposing agonist/antagonist muscle groups and aim for bilateral development of these groups.
- All equipment used should meet the standards set down for exercise equipment by the relevant bodies.
- Caution must be taken with resistance exercise involving the hyper-tension of the lower back and with exercises involving extreme joint flection.
- Finish with an adequate cool-down.
- Particular care should be given to a lifter with high blood pressure.
- Individual record cards should be available for lifters so that work-outs can be standardised and recorded.
- Regular monitoring of cards by the instructor should occur and this should be accompanied by regular consultations with the individual.
- Know the emergency procedure if a serious injury occurs.

Emergency procedure Although injuries are rare, a resistance-training facility should have an emergency procedure to deal with a serious injury that requires medical attention. The plan should be posted in the weights room and all instructors should be familiar with it. An emergency plan should include the following:

- a telephone number for the nearest ambulance service and/or hospital
- location of the nearest hospital or emergency room
- a complete first aid kit
- All instructors should have basic first aid and cardiopulmonary resuscitation (CPR) skills.

26 Complementary and Alternative Therapies

CONTRIBUTED BY JOHN W. BENEY

With the rapid development and popularity of naturo-pathic and holistic medicine, there are now many choices of natural health care available to the general public. Today's physical therapist needs to have a basic understanding of these quite diverse therapies, many with roots going back thousands of years and from every continent, others comparatively new and in the process of further development.

This chapter looks at:

- **acupuncture and Chinese medicine**
- **acupressure**
- **the Alexander technique**
- **aromatherapy**
- **Bach flower remedies and other flower essences**
- **chiropractic**
- **herbalism**
- **homeopathy**
- **osteopathy**
- **reflexology.**

Never before have we seen such a coming together of eastern and western medicine to offer clients a truly holistic alternative to pure allopathic medicine. But perhaps of greater importance to the therapist in private practice, he or she now has the opportunity to offer a complementary therapy that can work alone or alongside allopathic medicine.

It is estimated that in Europe, more than half of the population has used complementary therapy at some time and the majority of the medical profession is also interested in, if not using, complementary medicine. This chapter looks briefly at the more popular therapies and, by gaining a greater knowledge of their potential, you will be better able to refer clients to a suitable therapy compatible with their needs, outlook and beliefs.

Many complementary therapists believe that there is a life force, an electromagnetic energy. In China this life force is called *Chi* and in Japan, *Qi* and in India, *Prana*. This energy moves through channels called *meridians* and flows up the front channels and then down the back. If these channels become blocked for any reason, then discomfort and illness can ensue. The therapist's aim is to rebalance these energy channels, recreating good health.

Acupuncture and Chinese medicine

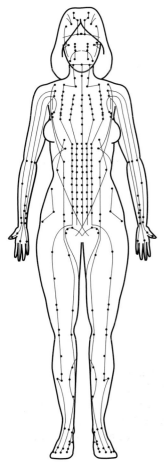

THE BASIC MERIDIANS AND
ACUPUNCTURE POINTS

Traditional Chinese medicine is a philosophy very different from the medical practices of the west and derives from an awareness of the laws of nature and the order of the universe. It is based on the Chinese belief that life is activated by the energy force *Chi* or *Qi*, which translated means life force or vital force. The amount and quality of *Chi* is determined partly by heredity, and how we live our lives also influences our *Chi*. We enhance our store of energy by taking care of ourselves, we add to our energy by eating the right foods, supporting it with proper exercise and the air we breathe.

The principle premise of Chinese medicine is that there are two opposing energy forces, *Yin* and *Yang*, which are present in every aspect of the universe, for example light and dark, cold and hot, good and evil, and good health is achieved through a balance between these opposing forces. The complexities of Chinese medicine include other principles such as the five elements, earth, fire, water, wood and metal, and the relationship between these and other elements serve to provide the practitioner with a reading of the deficiencies or imbalance of the patient.

Acupuncture is the most commonly known aspect of traditional Chinese medicine and may be used alone or as part of a complex system of treatment which could include herbal preparations, food therapy, exercise, and massage. The flow of energy, or *Chi*, is through the meridians, which are pathways around the body and each are linked to a particular organ or function of the body.

From the consultation the practitioner will determine which energy points may be sluggish or blocked and require attention. These points are stimulated by the insertion of very fine needles, sometimes with the application of heat, which is generated by burning *moxa*. The traditional moxa is made from the pressed and dried leaves of mugwort and the technique is called *moxibustion*.

The functions of the whole body, or just specific parts and systems, can be enhanced by acupuncture and regular treatments are considered a preventive medicine for creating and maintaining health. A comprehensive medical knowledge and training is required before graduating in this therapy.

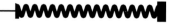

A TYPICAL CHINESE LOOP-TYPE DISPOSABLE ACUPUNCTURE NEEDLE

Acupressure

A number of massage techniques that use manual pressure to stimulate the energy points on the body come under the general description of acupressure. The therapist applies light or medium pressure with fingers to the same points used in acupuncture. The therapist may also use hands, feet, knees and elbows to stimulate these energy points.

The most well-known techniques of acupressure include *Shiatsu*, *Do-In*, *Jin Shin* and *Tui Na*, although there are many more, and variations are continually being evolved.

The purpose of this technique, as in acupuncture, is to stimulate the body's electromagnetic energy to assist the body's own recuperative powers to remove energy blockages. These blockages may be the result of the build-up of lactic acid and carbon monoxide in muscle tissue, causing the musculature to stiffen, putting pressures on the nervous and circulatory systems. These, in turn, adversely affect the functions of the internal organs. Removal of the blockages relaxes the whole body and helps to restore harmony to the systems.

The Alexander Technique

This technique was devised by the Australian actor, Frederick Alexander (born 1869), who discovered, as a result of his own periodic voice loss, that he had a habit of straining his neck and head when reciting. His discovery came about after careful self-observation over a number of years, studying his posture by looking at himself in mirrors and then by training himself to adopt a relaxed posture with his head held in its natural position in relation to his neck and torso, he found his vocal problem improved. However, he soon slipped back into bad habits and with the deterioration of his posture, so the vocal problems occurred again and eventually he trained himself to maintain the correct posture naturally.

He was so impressed he started to teach other actors, and again noted improvements, not only in their voices, but also in their general state of

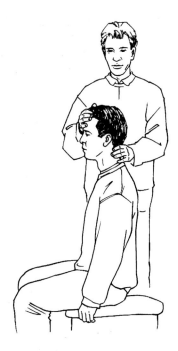

THE ALEXANDER TEACHER GUIDES THE PUPIL TO THE CORRECT POSTURE, GENTLY CHANGING MUSCLE TONE TO RELIEVE TENSIONS

health. He further developed the technique, to encompass the full range of bodily movements and posture and came to England at the turn of the century where he started to teach his technique.

Alexander conceived the technique as a series of lessons in which the teacher guides the pupil through a series of postural changes, aimed at demonstrating that there can be perfect balance and movement with the minimum of tension. Through the series of lessons, the pupil comes to understand the concept of the technique, increasing his or her awareness of posture and notices from the very first lesson improvements in his or her co-ordination of balance and movement. These improvements, in turn, affect body functioning.

Aromatherapy

Aromatherapy is the systematic use of essential oils in holistic treatments to improve physical and emotional well-being. Essential oils are extracted from plants, either from their leaves, flowers and roots, from woods, leaves and resins of trees and from the zest of citrus fruits. They are extracted in many ways, the most common being by steam distillation.

All the oils consist of many natural chemicals, most contain a few major ones, plus many trace elements which sometimes run into many hundreds and account for the therapeutic uses of the essential oils. For example, different oils work on the various body systems to restore *homoeostasis*, some work on emotional levels and all have antiseptic properties.

Essential oils can be used in very many ways: in a diffuser to perfume and disinfect the air, which both relaxes and prevents the spread of airborne infection, in lotions, soaps, bath oils, on tissues, in insect repellents. However by far the most effective way is by introducing the essential oils to the body by massage, as they are readily absorbed through the skin and the gentle physiological and psychological effects combine well to promote positive health. These oils must not be used neat, but mixed in a very low dilution with a base oil, such as Sweet Almond. Some of these oils are very powerful and only a trained aromatherapist should use them on clients.

On the psychological side, we know that our sense of smell works on a subconscious level, the olfactory nerves connect to the brain's limbic system, which also regulates sensory motor activities which affects many behavioural mechanisms.

In a similar way to herbs and homeopathic medicines, the same essential oil may be used to treat different conditions, due to its chemical constituents, whilst the same condition could respond well to more than one essential oil. This is very helpful where one particular odour may be disliked by a client, even though the oil would produce the beneficial therapeutic effect. So an alternative and equally suitable oil can be offered that is acceptable to the client.

Fifteen common essential oils

Bergamot	Chamomile	Eucalyptus
Geranium	Lavender	Lemon
Lemongrass	Mandarin	Neroli
Orange	Peppermint	Rose Otto
Rosemary	Sandalwood	Tea Tree

Forty essential oils for the professional aromatherapist

Basil	Bergamot	Benzoin	Black Pepper
Chamomile	Cedarwood	Cinnamon	Clary Sage
Clove	Cypress	Eucalyptus	Frankincense
Fennel (sweet)	Geranium	Ginger	Grapefruit
Jasmine	Juniper	Lavender	Lemon
Lemongrass	Mandarin	Marjoram	Melissa
Myrrh	Neroli	Naiouli	Orange (sweet)
Patchouli	Peppermint	Petitgrain	Pine
Rose Otto	Rosemary	Sandalwood	Tea Tree
Thyme	Valerian	Vetiver	Ylang Ylang

Essential oils were used many thousands of years ago by the Greeks, Romans, Indians and Chinese. Today there are many research programmes in progress, which are confirming that the traditional uses that have been passed down through the ages are scientifically correct.

Bach Flower Remedies and other flower essences

Bach Flower Therapy is the system of treatment in which a flower remedy is given to the client to act on their emotions, which are considered to be the place where the problem of a physical or other nature has originated.

In 1930 Dr Edward Bach, a prominent homeopath and bacteriologist, started a research programme to find a simple method of healing, being concerned about the side effects of drug therapy. He believed that nothing should be destroyed or changed and in the six years before his death, he developed the therapy that now bears his name. Bach believed that the unique healing power of a plant is in its energetic property. This is a holistic concept used by many other therapists and the thought is that if they become disconnected, stress and then disease can set in. Dr Bach developed 38 flower remedies to treat various emotional problems. The flower essences are taken by mouth and usually a few drops are placed under the tongue and can be administered up to four times a day. The essences can then be used individually or in combination. For example, the famous 'Rescue Remedy', that many people always carry with them, is a combination of five different essences and can be used to counter the effects of shock, during or after an emergency or stressful experience.

Flower essence is a general term for a liquid preparation created by immersing a flower into water and exposing the preparation to sunlight or heat. This process brings out healing properties and spiritual elements contained in the flower. This infusion is called the 'mother stock', which is diluted with brandy and is ready for general use.

Just as we consume food to nourish or use herbs to heal the physical body, flower remedies and essences are used to nourish, as well as help heal the physical body. According to developers of flower preparations, these products strengthen the individual and allow his or her innate spiritual powers to enhance the body and the mind's natural healing abilities. Bach Remedies are included in the homeopathic pharmacopoeia.

In more recent years, many other flower essences and products have been developed around the world, each system having a different focus which gives the therapist a wide range of options and choice.

The 38 Bach Flower Remedies

Remedy	Helpful for people who:
Agrimony	hide their feelings behind a brave face
Aspen	have unknown fears which fill them with panic for no apparent reason
Beech	find it difficult to understand the shortcomings of others
Centaury	find it hard to stand up for themselves
Cerato	distrust their own judgement
Cherry plum	have a fear of insanity
Chestnut bud	cannot learn the lessons of life
Chicory	are of a 'mothering' type
Clematis	lack interest in the present because their minds are full of the future
Crab apple	feel they have been soiled (a cleansing remedy)
Elm	find the burden of their responsibility becomes too heavy to bear
Gentian	are despondent and discouraged, as a result of disappointment
Gorse	whose despondency turns to despair and they become forlorn
Heather	are chatterboxes with total self-absorption with their troubles
Holly	are jealous, envious, and full of hatred, revenge, suspicion
Honeysuckle	dwell on memories of life gone by, regrets of missed opportunities
Hornbeam	need emotional strength to face the day ahead
Impatiens	are impatient and irritable
Larch	lack confidence in themselves
Mimulus	have a fear of known things – fear of illness, the fears of everyday life
Mustard	suffer depression which descends like a dark cloud
Oak	are the fighters but eventually find their strength is no longer there
Olive	are so drained of energy that they feel too tired to go on
Pine	have feelings of guilt (which may stem from the past or more recent)
Red chestnut	are afraid of something happening to their loved ones
Rock rose	suffer extreme fear and panic which is not always rational
Rock water	are self-righteous and generally enjoy their stringent lifestyle
Scleranthus	suffer emotional distress through indecision
Star of Bethlehem	suffer shock due to trauma to the system
Sweet chestnut	suffer desperate mental anguish and feelings of utter despair
Vervain	have strong principles (helps them to wind down and relax)
Vine	are self-assured, dominant (the leaders and rulers)
Walnut	have difficulty settling into a new environment
Water violet	stand proud and erect
White chestnut	whose mind is tormented by worrying and unwanted thoughts
Wild oat	have come to life's crossroads and don't know which way to go
Wild rose	are inclined to become apathetic and resigned to all that happens
Willow	have become so introspective that they dwell on their misfortune

Chiropractic

Chiropractic has been defined as an independent branch of medicine concerned with the diagnosis and treatment of mechanical disorders of joints, particularly spinal joints and their effects on the nervous system. Diagnosis may include the use of X-rays and the treatment is done mostly by hand without the use of drugs or surgery. Chiropractors may therefore be considered spinal specialists who believe that many of the problems relating to the spine are caused from misalignments or maladjustments and excess strain placed on the intervertebral joints.

Manipulative treatment was known in the days of the ancient Greek physician, Hypocrites, some 2500 years ago, and it was the work of Canadian born Daniel Palmer, just before the turn of the century, that reintroduced the therapy as chiropractic is known today.

The term *sublaxation* is used by chiropractors to describe the condition of bones which are out of alignment, and it is this condition that gives rise to restricted mobility or excessive mobility. It is believed the energy transmitted from the brain to the bodily organs through the spinal cord can be affected by the pressure on the nerve leaving the misaligned vertebrae which can cause irritation or excitation, which may either increase the nerve force or reduce the flow of energy.

Manipulative therapies such as chiropractic are necessary to realign the skeletal system when sublaxation becomes obvious and, while the traditional use of chiropractic is principally confined to spinal manipulation, the more popular view is that chiropractic encompasses every health care tool except drugs and surgery. The blockage or reduction of the energy flow, as we have seen earlier, affects the functions of the internal organs and the realignment of the vertebrae and release of the energy blockage helps to restore a healthy equilibrium or homeostasis.

Herbalism

Herbalism is a therapeutic system based on the use of herbs, sometimes taken as teas, in the treatment of a wide range of ailments.

The use of plant materials is as old as civilisation, with every known culture using local flora for medicinal and nutritional purposes. Knowledge of the plants' medical powers was handed down from generation to generation and eventually people began to write down their findings, recording details of which herbs had been successfully used for which illness.

Herbalism is known as the 'art of simpling'. Herbs were known as *simples* because one herb can cure many different conditions. Herbal medicines are believed to work biochemically in the body and taken in moderate doses for long enough, these biochemical responses become automatic, even after one stops taking the herbs.

When used in medical treatments, herbs have three functions:

- to detoxify the body and to eliminate waste
- to strengthen the body to help it heal itself
- to build up the organs

233

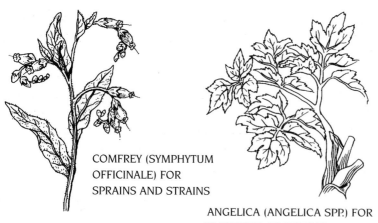

COMFREY (SYMPHYTUM OFFICINALE) FOR SPRAINS AND STRAINS

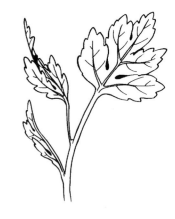

ANGELICA (ANGELICA SPP.) FOR BRONCHIAL PROBLEMS

MUGWORT (ARTEMISIA VULGARIS), A GENTLE NERVINE

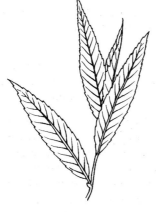

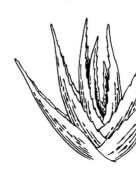

WILLOW (SALIX ALBA) FOR ARTHRITIS AND RHEUMATISM

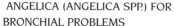

ALOE (ALOE VERA) FOR FUNGAL INFECTIONS

Three basic principles should be considered when selecting herbal remedies:

- The types of disease found in a certain geographical area to some extent depend on the environmental conditions of that area and so herbs that grow in a particular area may well treat the problems contracted in it.
- Only mild herbs should be used because they can then be taken freely and have a gentle effect on the body.
- A high dose of these mild herbs may be used in order to produce the required effect.

Herbs are categorised according to their effects on the body, which are stimulation, tranquilisation, blood purification, tonification, diuresis, sweating, emesis and purging.

There are many systems for using herbs. English herbalists tend to use single herbs for a specific ailment or condition, whilst the Chinese will make their herbal prescriptions in carefully formulated combinations to achieve more general effects and benefits.

It has been mentioned that herbs are sometimes taken as teas, but there are many ways to use herbal remedies and these may include:

- *capsules* and *tablets*, which are taken by mouth
- *decoctions*, in which the herbs are boiled down into a thick concentrate and strained

- *inhalation*, in which streamed or atomised fluids are breathed in
- *herbal baths*, in which absorption takes place through skin pores or lungs via steam
- *tinctures/linaments*, in which herbal essences are infused in alcohol
- *ointments, salves, lotions, and oils*, in which the herbal properties are infused into oil
- *infusion*, in which more delicate herbs are steeped in boiling water
- *tisane*, in which various parts of plants are brewed into a tea
- *mastication*, in which bark, roots, or leaves are chewed.

Homeopathy

The principles of homeopathy have been known since the time of the ancient Greeks – Hippocrates made mention of 'similars' in his early writings. It is a system of medicine based on the theory of 'like cures like'.

The name *homeopathy* was first used by the German doctor Samuel Hahnemann in his *Homeopathic Meteria Medica*, published in the early 1800s and this was the beginning of homeopathy as we know it today.

It was much earlier, in the late 1700s that Dr Hahnemann, dissatisfied with the medical procedures of the day, started his research, having already discovered that the taking of a small dose of quinine by a healthy person produced the symptoms of malaria. He treated people in a holistic way and developed many remedies after practising on himself and others. He believed the agents that cause the symptoms of sickness in a healthy person can cure the cause of those same symptoms in an unhealthy person, when used in extreme dilution.

Homeopathic preparations or remedies are essences of natural substances derived from plants, animal materials, and natural chemicals.

Homeopathic philosophy is based on the belief that symptoms are signs of the body's effort to throw off disease; one must treat the cause of the disease and not the symptoms. As with many other therapies, the homeopath believes in the body's own ability to heal itself.

Osteopathy

The word *osteo* means to do with bones. Osteopathy was first developed by an American called Andrew Still. He was a mechanic and, following the death of his three children from meningitis, he started to think about why people became ill. He thought that like machinery, if the structure of the body was out of alignment, then sickness followed. In 1892 he started a school of osteopathy.

John Martin Littlejohn enrolled at Still's school. He had previously studied physiology in Glasgow. With his knowledge of physiology and with Still's mechanical theories, they developed a treatment called the Science of Adjustment. This was looked upon as a holistic therapy.

Osteopathy was developed before chiropractic and today in America is practised alongside orthodox medicine. In Britain it is recognised and practised both in private clinics and within the National Health Service.

Before one can train to be an osteopath one has to have completed a recognised medical training followed by 500 hours studying the body's structure, particularly the skeletal and muscular systems. Students learn how to examine, treat and to recognise abnormalities. They also learn how to prescribe medication of both herbal and prescription drugs.

Students of osteopathy are taught that the principles of healing are that the body contains its own self-healing mechanisms and that these work best when there is maximum mobility and flexibility. To treat the body as a whole and that disorder in one area will negatively affect other areas. They work on the spine and the nerves travelling towards and away from the spine and to the different organs that they supply. They believe the disease can be caused by damage along the nerve pathways and that this is worse when the nerves pass through bones. Incorrect impulses are then transmitted along the fibres. Posture is considered to be an important healing factor and also the position of joints. They learn a technique of soft tissue massage, stretching and a special joint manipulation to release joint fixations.

Dr Still, along with many other natural therapists, taught his students to look firstly for the cause of problems before treating the symptoms.

Back pain is a major part of the work of osteopaths, but many other disturbances belonging to other systems are treated. Cranial osteopathy specialises in head problems, especially those arising from birth injuries in babies and children.

Reflexology

In ancient times when feet were our main method of transport, they were revered very much more than they are today. Feet were washed, stroked and massaged. There are many references to their importance in the Bible.

Work on the feet has a history which has been passed down through the ages and practised by many cultures. In Egypt, in the tomb of Ankhmahor the physician, wall carvings were found showing work being done on the feet. From China there is a picture showing this being practised in 1870.

The science and art of *reflexology* as we know it today was developed by Eunice Ingham in America during the 1930s. Her theory was that the body is divided into ten energy zones running the length of the body, and if there are blockages within these pathways there is dysfunction within the body. After many years of experience, she devised foot charts showing the precise positions of the body's anatomy.

The science works on the principal that there are reflex points in both the feet and the hands that relate to all organs and body systems. These are linked to the ten energy zones through our natural electrical impulses.

When working on the feet, the thumb and finger pressures stimulate these energies through the thousands of nerve endings within the feet, this stimulation will help to restore the body to a state of *homeostasis*.

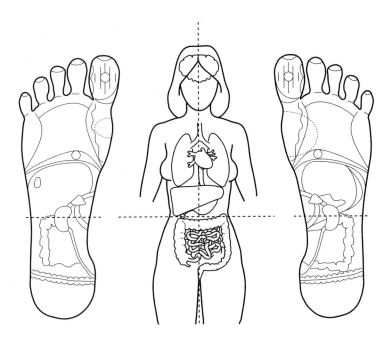

THE ORGANS OF THE BODY ARE
MIRRORED IN THE FEET

Reflexology has been found to:

- help the body's own healing process
- encourage the general circulation
- help to eliminate toxins from the body
- stimulate the digestive and urinary systems.

Emotionally it also seems to restore balance, is relaxing, reduces stress levels and helps to restore sleep patterns for those suffering with insomnia.

The reflexologist uses massage initially, then a walking technique with the thumbs and fingers. Reflexology should not be painful to the client and in time both the therapist and the client become more sensitive to touch, and health problems show up on the feet – these may be current problems or even disorders from the past.

Hands can be worked the same way, particularly useful if the foot has been contra-indicated, and this technique is ideal for self-help.

Management of Patient and Practice

The preceding chapters have been devoted to providing the knowledge necessary to undertake treatments. In other words, an understanding of the body and how it works; what may go wrong with it and how physical therapy may accelerate those physiological processes necessary for the body to return to a state of normality and health.

The physical therapist is, however, a professional person and this involves much more than just the knowledge and expertise acquired from basic training. The following section endeavours to fill in some of those gaps and to help you to become a responsible, successful member of an honourable profession.

27 Patient Assessment

The physical therapist's assessment of a patient is very important and it is equally important to record that assessment correctly. A good therapist learns how to observe accurately and to note any abnormality. Observation in this sense is not only done by means of the eyes, but with the nose, ear and hand. The nose will detect any unusual odour, for example, diabetes is sometimes associated with sweet smelling breath which will enable the therapist to take the necessary precautions in treatment, especially heat treatments. The ear will detect any unusual breathing sound and panting or bronchitic breathing will make the therapist proceed with extreme caution. Also, when massaging the patient the fingers should be taught to automatically flash back to the brain anything unusual in the body structure, a protuberance that does not correspond to a normal anatomical one, or a rise in temperature on a particular part of the skin suggesting inflammation, or increased sensitivity. When such abnormalities are found they must be referred back to the patient's medical adviser before treatment of the part is undertaken.

You will note that this chapter is headed 'Patient Assessment' and that the word 'diagnosis' is not used. Diagnosis is the province of the properly qualified medical person.

Patient records

Assuming that the patient has already been given an assessment, or alternatively that they are coming in for general treatment such as toning or relaxation treatment, then it is necessary to record the patient's requirements, and certainly in the case of slimming treatment it is necessary to have certain statistical records. These records must, of

241

necessity, vary according to the type of clinic or practice in which you are involved as the following two examples show:

- Example of the type of patient information that would be recorded in a clinic which provides slimming support treatments:

  date, name, address, telephone number, age, sex, reason for coming, therapist's observations and on the other side of the card in vertical columns: date, height, weight, bust, waist, abdomen, hips, thighs and a blank column

- Example of the type of patient information that would be recorded in a clinic which has numerous medical referrals:

  date, name, address, telephone number, age, sex, occupation, name of doctor, brief medical history, what drugs have been taken and for how long, therapist's observations.

The information required in the first example could easily be put on an index card, whilst the second one requires a larger card or index sheet

Points to note when making an assessment

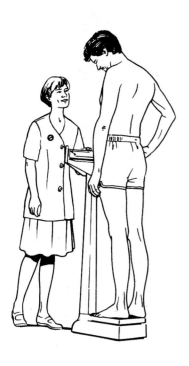

The patient should be weighed either in the nude or with a minimum of clothing. The first reason for this is that the weight of the clothing can easily alter from visit to visit. Secondly, observing the patient in a state of undress enables the therapist to see more clearly the body structure, posture, large fat folds, etc. Weighing is not normally recommended more than once a week and it should preferably be done at the same time of the day. In the case of the female patient, allowance should be made for the monthly cycle because many women put on extra weight (due to water retention) in the immediate premenstrual part of the cycle. Their weight can go up as much as 2–3 kg, though the average increase is probably 1 kg.

As a guide, the tables opposite show the *maximum* desirable weight relative to height and frame. All the weights given are for the naked body. The tables are based on those of life assurance companies.

The formula for establishing the frame category is as follows:

Take the width of the ribs laterally (in the axilla region) and the width of the hips laterally at the widest point. Add these together, multiply by 2 and add 13 for women or 19 for men. If this total approximately equals the height in inches, this is a *medium* frame. If the total is two or more inches less than the height, then the frame is *small*. Two or more inches greater and the frame is *large*. A pelvimeter which is normally used for determining pelvic size is an excellent instrument for taking these measurements.

Measurements should be taken with the tape just snugly fitting over the part being measured, not tight enough to create an indentation in the fat nor loose enough for the tape to sag. With practice the right amount of tightness can be achieved so avoiding the very common error of false measurements.

Maximum weight desirable for women

Height		Small frame		Medium frame		Large frame	
4′ 11″	1.50 m	7 st. 4 lb	46.3 kg	7 st. 13 lb	50.3 kg	8 st. 11 lb	55.8 kg
5′ 0″	1.52 m	7 st. 5 lb	47.7 kg	8 st. 2 lb	51.7 kg	9 st. 0 lb	57.1 kg
5′ 1″	1.55 m	7 st. 10 lb	49.0 kg	8 st. 5 lb	53.0 kg	9 st. 3 lb	58.5 kg
5′ 2″	1.57 m	7 st. 13 lb	50.3 kg	8 st. 9 lb	54.9 kg	9 st. 7 lb	60.3 kg
5′ 3″	1.60 m	8 st. 2 lb	51.7 kg	8 st. 13 lb	56.7 kg	9 st. 11 lb	62.1 kg
5′ 4″	1.63 m	8 st. 6 lb	53.4 kg	9 st. 4 lb	59.0 kg	10 st. 1 lb	63.9 kg
5′ 5″	1.65 m	8 st. 10 lb	55.3 kg	9 st. 10 lb	61.7 kg	10 st. 5 lb	65.8 kg
5′ 6″	1.68 m	9 st. 0 lb	57.1 kg	9 st. 12 lb	62.6 kg	10 st. 9 lb	67.6 kg
5′ 7″	1.70 m	9 st. 4 lb	59.0 kg	10 st. 2 lb	64.4 kg	10 st. 13 lb	69.4 kg
5′ 8″	1.73 m	9 st. 9 lb	61.2 kg	10 st. 6 lb	66.2 kg	11 st. 4 lb	71.5 kg
5′ 9″	1.75 m	9 st. 13 lb	63.0 kg	10 st. 10 lb	67.9 kg	11 st. 9 lb	73.8 kg
5′ 10″	1.78 m	10 st. 3 lb	64.9 kg	11 st. 0 lb	69.7 kg	12 st. 1 lb	76.7 kg

Maximum weight desirable for men

Height		Small frame		Medium frame		Large frame	
5′ 3″	1.60 m	8 st. 6 lb	53.4 kg	9 st. 2 lb	58.0 kg	10 st. 0 lb	63.5 kg
5′ 4″	1.63 m	8 st. 9 lb	54.9 kg	9 st. 5 lb	59.4 kg	10 st. 4 lb	65.3 kg
5′ 5″	1.65 m	8 st. 13 lb	56.7 kg	9 st. 9 lb	61.2 kg	10 st. 8 lb	67.2 kg
5′ 6″	1.68 m	9 st. 3 lb	58.5 kg	9 st. 13 lb	63.0 kg	10 st. 13 lb	69.4 kg
5′ 7″	1.70 m	9 st. 7 lb	60.3 kg	10 st. 4 lb	65.3 kg	11 st. 4 lb	71.5 kg
5′ 8″	1.73 m	9 st. 11 lb	62.1 kg	10 st. 8 lb	67.2 kg	11 st. 8 lb	73.3 kg
5′ 9″	1.75 m	10 st. 2 lb	64.4 kg	10 st. 12 lb	69.0 kg	11 st. 12 lb	75.2 kg
5′ 10″	1.78 m	10 st. 6 lb	66.2 kg	11 st. 3 lb	71.1 kg	12 st. 3 lb	77.5 kg
5′ 11″	1.80 m	10 st. 10 lb	67.9 kg	11 st. 8 lb	73.3 kg	12 st. 8 lb	79.9 kg
6′ 0″	1.83 m	11 st. 0 lb	69.7 kg	11 st. 11 lb	74.8 kg	12 st. 13 lb	82.3 kg
6′ 1″	1.85 m	11 st. 5 lb	72.1 kg	12 st. 2 lb	77.1 kg	13 st. 4 lb	86.2 kg
6′ 2″	1.88 m	11 st. 9 lb	73.8 kg	12 st. 7 lb	79.4 kg	13 st. 9 lb	88.4 kg
6′ 3″	1.90 m	11 st. 11 lb	74.8 kg	13 st. 0 lb	82.6 kg	14 st. 0 lb	90.7 kg

In noting the medical history (this is normally limited to those conditions likely to be affected by physical therapy), take particular note of operations, accidents and cardio-vascular troubles. If the patient volunteers the information that he or she is taking drugs or other medications, find out which ones, why and for how long.

When a patient comes specifically for slimming support treatment it is useful to note whether he or she is currently on a diet, has been on a diet in the past or has never been on a diet. It might also be worth noting whether the patient has been overweight since childhood, puberty, marriage, first child or menopause in the case of a female or, in the case of a male, since the age of approximately 20, 30, 40 or 50.

Under the heading 'occupation' many are self-explanatory and give a good idea as to whether the patient is likely to be standing for most of the day or sitting for most of the day with a lot or little exercise. When a patient puts an occupation such as 'housewife' it might be worthwhile exploring her other activities to find out whether she plays golf, walks, gardens, rides, etc.

Under the heading 'reason for coming' it is usual to note any special instructions which the doctor may have given.

Finally, either on the case history sheet or, more usually, on a separate card, a record must be kept of the patient's attendances, the dates, the treatment being received on those dates and the amount paid or to be charged.

The above ideas are given purely as guides. They indicate the kind of information required and should enable you to produce a case history sheet or card index particularly appropriate to your type of practice or clinic. Whichever form is finally adopted, it cannot be over-emphasised that the keeping of adequate records is an integral part of professional life.

28 Clinic Organisation and Management

This chapter is aimed at helping newly qualified therapists in the course of setting up a practice or those who are expecting to occupy a position of management in someone else's employment.

It is stressed that rules and regulations vary from country to country, state to state and even county to county. It is therefore important to regard this chapter as a general guide rather than a statement of facts. It should, however, help you to identify the main areas in which advice needs to be obtained from a professional or from the local authority.

Premises

Planning consent
Having located premises which appear suitable for the purpose of establishing a clinic, it should be ascertained whether consent has been given for the purpose to which they are to be put. In the UK, this comes under the Planning Department of the local town or district council – there are offices in most large centres of population. In most other countries there are similar bodies.

Business name
Following a change in the law in early 1982 it is no longer necessary to register a business name. All that is required (when the name under which the business is trading is not your own personal name) is that the name of the business plus the name and address of the owner must be put on to a card and placed where it may easily be seen by persons visiting the premises.

Licence to practice and registration
Most countries require a licence to practise and information about this may be obtained from the Department of Health, Medical Officers of Health, Department of Public Control or Department of the Environment. In the UK, application is normally made to the Chief Trading Standards Officer or the Environmental Health Officer who can advise you of their requirements for the area. The usual stipulation is that you should have graduated from a college or training centre

recognised by the Department and/or have an internationally-recognised qualification, such as ITEC. The licence granted will only be for work within the areas for which you have documentary evidence of proficiency. The principal areas of treatment are:

- massage
- heat treatments (including sauna)
- electrical treatments
- ultraviolet ray treatments.

The authority will indicate what controls they have on advertising, the publications of prices, requirements for safety, electrical checks and fire precautions and they may, at their discretion, impose limits on the therapies practised. For example, the authorities may refuse to include sauna treatments in the licence because of the unsuitability of the building. When a licence has been granted, it is normally renewable yearly and the practice is subject to inspection at any normal time to enable the inspector to ascertain whether it is being run strictly within the terms prescribed by the licence.

Premises on which epilation or ear piercing is carried out have to be registered in the UK and are subject to inspection. Some authorities require an annual certificate of safety from a qualified electrician, but in any case it is advisable for regular safety checks to be made on equipment, especially where electricity is concerned.

Insurance When the licence has been obtained and before accepting the first patient, the premises and its contents should be insured including third party indemnity. This is to cover accidents other than those arising out of the treatments, for example, if a person visiting the premises falls down the stairs. Additionally, you must have professional public indemnity insurance. This is protection against accidents or injury happening to the patient during the course of treatment and this cover will normally be obtained through the professional body of which you are a member.

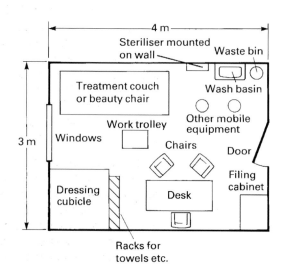

EXAMPLE OF LAYOUT OF A
CONSULTING ROOM DOUBLING
UP FOR TREATMENT

Clinic facilities The premises are expected to have reasonable toilet and washing facilities for both staff and patients, the provision of a first aid box, fire extinguisher(s) and a free-standing or wall thermometer to indicate that the heating is at a satisfactory level.

Setting up a practice

Costs Practices fall generally into two categories:

- visiting only
- clinic.

Before embarking on setting up either type it is important to estimate the costs involved. These can be classified as follows:

- *capital expenditure* – purchase and preparation of premises (or car), equipment, etc.
- *overheads of the premises* – including business rates, rent (if rented or leased property), light, heat, cleaning, laundry, etc.
- *expendables* – tissues, paper towels, cosmetics, magazines for waiting room, etc.
- *labour* – including an allowance for yourself
- *publicity* – brochures, price lists, advertising and other public relations
- *professional services* – e.g. accountant, solicitor.

Capital expenditure is going to be the largest outgoing and for the purposes of preparing an estimate, it should be broken down over a period of five years. All other costs are recurring and should be allowed for.

The possible income generated must be offset against the costs and this is where many new practitioners make mistakes. Although you may be prepared to work eight hours a day, six days a week, 50 weeks a year, it would be foolish to assume that the whole of that time would be filled up with clients. First you have to build up a list of clients, but even when this has been achieved you will find many blanks in your appointment book due to clients' holidays, illness (of clients themselves or their dependants) and even bad weather. Established practitioners are well aware of this situation, but you should not overlook it when starting out. The risk is reduced in a visiting practice, but here allowances must be made for travelling time.

If you do not have sufficient personal capital to start a practice, equipment may be purchased on a hire purchase agreement or a loan may be obtained from the bank or building society, but in each of these cases the interest can amount to a large sum and must be allowed for. When borrowing money, especially on hire purchase, it is easy to be influenced by salesmen to buy equipment which is not absolutely essential to the efficient running of the practice. Remember, it is easy to buy additional equipment when current equipment is justifying itself or when new demands arise.

Publicity You will need a leaflet or brochure setting out your services. This should be concise, include your name, address, telephone number and of course your qualifications. If you are running a clinic, the hours of business should be stated, and if the practice is a visiting one, the area of operation should be given. Reference should be made to any specialities you practise and it is a good idea to give some indication of costs, at least for your basic treatments. For example:

Full facial (1 hour)	....
Body massage (1 hour)	....
Sports clinic (½ hour treatment)	....

These brochures should be distributed as widely as possible locally.

Large advertisements in the press rarely justify the cost, except possibly for special occasions like an opening. However a regular small advertisement in the personal or medical services column of the local weekly paper will keep your name, address and telephone number constantly before the public.

If you are working on your own, an answering machine is a good investment. Your recorded message should be short and to the point and should say that you will phone back as soon as you are free.

National Insurance Whether you are working for yourself or in a partnership you will have to pay a Class II stamp on a weekly basis. This applies to the UK, but other countries have comparable systems.

Value Added Tax (VAT) Each year the Chancellor of the Exchequer sets a minimum annual turnover figure for businesses and when the turnover of a particular business exceeds this figure, all its services and products become VAT rated. This means that VAT (at a set percentage rate) is added to their cost. Since the 1990 UK budget, liability is calculated in retrospect, i.e. on the turnover of the previous year. If a business is registered for VAT, the amount of VAT paid on goods or services bought from other companies can be claimed back from the government.

PAYE Pay-as-you-earn (PAYE) in the UK is a statutory system by which the employer is required to deduct the income tax at the time the wages or salary are paid. Each employee will have a P45 form from the previous employer and this form will show the employee's code number, the total remuneration to date and the amount of tax deducted. When the employee leaves your service he or she must be given an updated P45.

Accounts For tax purposes it is obligatory to keep accounts and in most countries tax laws are so complex it is advisable to employ an accountant, at least for the preparation of the yearly statement for submission to the Inspector of Taxes. The accountant will usually indicate the kind of records he or she wishes to be kept but, in the absence of such instructions or if the practice commences before an accountant is appointed, it is essential to keep a record of all monies received and paid out. In the case of the outgoings, they should be supported as far as possible by receipted bills or statements with a clear indication of the purpose for which the money was spent. Many expenses are subject to tax relief; in addition to the more obvious ones of rent, light, heat and telephone there are such recurring charges as laundry, cleaning, petrol and car expenses if the practice is a visiting one, provision of magazines for a waiting room and so on. If in doubt as to whether an item is eligible for tax relief or not, include it in your list and leave it to the professional accountant to eliminate it in the event of its being an inadmissible expense. The accountant will also advise you on VAT liability and how to operate the PAYE scheme if you have any employees. If you sell products of any kind you are also expected to have a simple form of stock control.

Contract of employment

The following information is given only as a guide to the regulations applying in the UK and generally in the countries of the EU. It is not intended to be comprehensive and if in any doubt please seek professional assistance. Other countries will have their own laws and information about these should be available locally.

If you employ staff you are required to give each employee a written statement of the terms of employment and this must be done within 13 weeks of the commencement of work. Such a statement must include the following:

- the names of employer and employee
- date when employment began
- scale of remuneration (or method of calculating it)
- whether payment is weekly or monthly
- terms and conditions relating to hours of work
- holiday arrangements
- procedures relating to sickness and injury
- length of notice required by either side
- job title.

Dismissal

An employee who has been employed for more than one month but less than two years is entitled to one week's notice. If employed continuously for more than two but less than 12 years, the entitlement is one week for each continuous year of service. For an employee with over 12 years' service not less than 12 weeks notice is required. *Unfair dismissal* is a complex subject which requires legal assistance.

Maternity leave

This is applicable to employees who have been in continuous employment for at least two years by the eleventh week before confinement.

Equipment

Specialised equipment has been dealt with in Part 2 of this book, but there is certain basic equipment which is common to most clinics and the following information should help you to choose that which is most appropriate to the type of practice envisaged.

Couches

Couches come in a variety of forms:

- the *lightweight* or *examination couch* This normally has a tilt head and is suitable for most treatments other than massage or manipulation. This is because the legs are bolted on to the frame and not cross supported.

- *massage couch* This usually has legs fitted as an integral part of the couch and cross struts to strengthen the legs. It costs rather more but is very much more substantial. Its height is usually 66 cm (26 inches) against the 76 cm (30 inches) of an examination couch. It is also fitted with a tilt head.

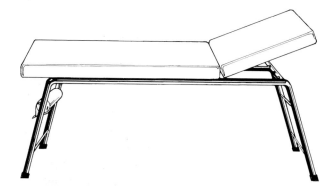

A MASSAGE COUCH WITH
TILT HEAD

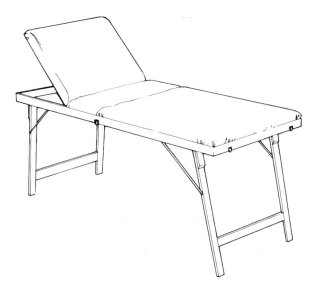

A FOLDING MASSAGE COUCH

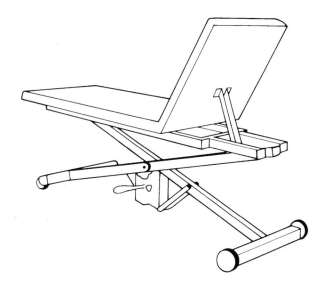

A HYDRAULIC COUCH

- the *folding massage couch* for therapists with visiting practices. This is very strong, is available with a tilt head and when folded will fit into the boot of most small cars.

- the *hydraulic couch* for the more sophisticated clinic. This is a very heavily built couch fitted with hydraulic lift, having a maximum height of about 90 cm (36 inches) and a minimum of 50 cm (19 inches). It is constructed from heavy gauge metal, the top being covered with expanded vinyl. The head has a multi-positional tilt.

- the *electric lift couch* – the ultimate in couches. It has a tilt head and, if required, a tilt foot and a cut-out section for the patient's nose when in a prone position. The couch can be supplied with a drop down undercarriage which enables it to be moved about.

For the therapist requiring a combination unit there is the '*Chouch*'. This is mounted on a tubular metal base and is designed so that it can be used as a treatment chair with an adjustable back and leg rest or, with the removal of the arms, as a level massage couch.

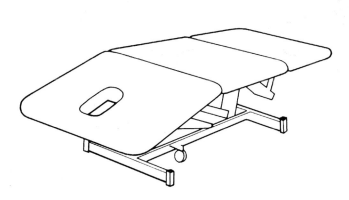

AN ELECTRIC LIFT COUCH

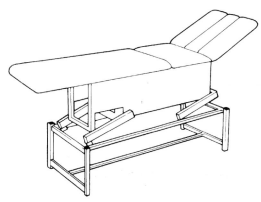

AN ELECTRIC MANIPULATION COUCH

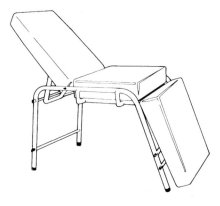

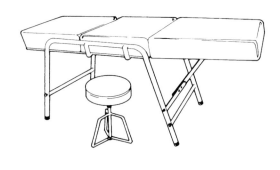

A 'CHOUCH' (COMBINED TREATMENT
COUCH AND CHAIR)

A 'CHOUCH' IN MASSAGE POSITION

Treatment trolleys These are available in a variety of models; the simplest one has two glass shelves. They are also available with guard rails to prevent instruments from sliding off the back and sides, and with drawers and cupboards. Usual sizes are 46 × 46 cm (18 inches × 18 inches), 61 × 46 cm (24 inches × 18 inches) and 76 × 46 × 86 cm (30 inches × 18 inches × 34 inches) high.

Scales Most therapists will be satisfied with low level, large dial scales; these are comparatively inexpensive in comparison with the more accurate sliding cursor scales which are available, if required, with height measures.

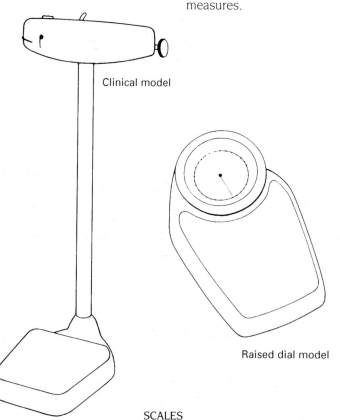

Clinical model

Raised dial model

SCALES

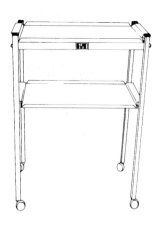

A TREATMENT TROLLEY

Sterilisers Cabinet sterilisers suitable for a physical therapy clinic come in two forms:

- the *vapour* type which is the cheaper
- the *ultraviolet ray* type.

The latter is suitable for keeping in a sterile condition instruments which have already been cleansed.

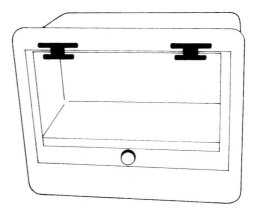

A CABINET STERILISER

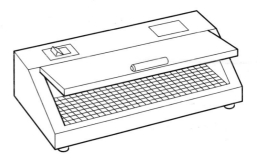

AN ULTRAVIOLET STERILISER

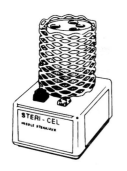

A BEAD STERILISER

Where invasive techniques are involved, e.g. electrolysis, particular care has to be taken to avoid infection especially hepatitis and HIV (human immunodeficiency virus). Here ordinary sterilising methods are not sufficient. It is therefore recommended that disposable needles be used. Otherwise needles should be autoclaved or put into a glass-bead type steriliser for a minimum of 20 minutes.

HIV

Outside of the body HIV is easily destroyed by normal disinfectants. The danger occurs when it enters the body via cuts, broken skin or body fluids. If a person who you know is HIV-positive or who is suffering from AIDS is being treated, in addition to the usual hygiene techniques it is suggested that disposable gloves be worn and disposable towels used. On the termination of the treatment those should be put into a sealed plastic bag. In addition, all contact surfaces should be thoroughly sterilised.

It is emphasised that the wearing of gloves does not apply to normal body treatments, but for invasive techniques only, such as epilation, and in dealing with injuries which are bleeding.

Towels   Towels are required for the couch and for patient use and there should be an adequate supply, allowing for laundry time. Paper towels to go on the couch are also available and these will save laundry bills as well as giving an ultra-hygienic appearance.

Gowns   Gowns are generally made from absorbent towelling material and may be purchased in the same colour as the towels.

Summary

- Do not enter into any binding agreement regarding property until you have first ascertained that planning consent has been given.
- Do not agree to purchase property until it has been professionally surveyed.
- Do not enter into partnership or similar arrangements before taking legal advice.

Professional help may appear expensive at the beginning of a career but it can save a lot of money and headaches later on.

29 Professionalism, Ethics and Patient Support

Professionalism, ethics and support form an important framework for a successful relationship between a therapist and his or her patient.

Professionalism

It is true to say that a therapist is, in fact, two persons – he or she is a private *and* a professional person, and the two are indivisible. A doctor is not only a doctor when he is working in a hospital or his surgery but is equally a representative of his profession when he is taking part in sport or leisure activities.

Professionalism is something that is acquired during the long period of training and it is a quality which becomes more marked when graduates have the responsibility of their own patients. There is no quick way of learning professionalism but there are some guidelines to help:

- When with a patient give that patient your undivided attention.
- Cultivate the art of putting out of your mind your own personal interests or problems.
- Forget about the previous patient and just concentrate on the present one.
- When the next patient is presented, make sure that you do not carry over problems from previous sessions.
- Always wear a white coat or other professional uniform and if you are a member of a professional body wear your membership badge. The uniform does more than protect your own clothes – it projects a professional image.
- Whether visiting or in your own clinic, always make a point of washing your hands before undertaking treatment and, if possible, do this in such a way that the patient is aware that you have done so.
- Never let a patient dictate the treatment nor the form it should take because you are the person who has the necessary knowledge to decide this, though it is reasonable to take the patient's preferences into account.
- Talk to the patient but do not gossip.
- Guard against any emotional involvement. This applies not only to problems relating to sex but a whole range of problems which may harass a patient. Give good, sound advice, help with the problem in any way you can, but do not become emotionally involved in it.

255

Ethics

The following extracts culled from the published code of ethics of two professional bodies indicate very clearly the standard of behaviour which is required from their professionally qualified members.

'Members shall, at all times, conduct their professional lives with the propriety and dignity becoming to a servant of the public and pledge that they will, at all times, place service before self. They also pledge that they will, under no circumstances, infringe the code of morality becoming to their profession and to commit no breach of conduct which will bring grief upon themselves, upon society or upon their fellow practitioners.'

'Members shall confine their services to within recognised spheres of their profession and shall not offer nor promise cures for specific conditions.'

'No member, who having been employed by a therapist, shall on leaving his employ attempt to persuade his former employer's patient to become his patients.'

'No member or Associate who is not a registered Medical Practitioner shall accept patients for medical diagnosis or for the treatment of a medical condition except on reference by a registered Medical Practitioner.'

'All members incur an obligation to uphold the dignity of the profession and they shall at all times act honourably towards their clients and fellow practitioners. They shall at all times maintain professional secrecy and shall refrain from criticising the work of a fellow practitioner.'

To these might be added three practices which are generally accepted:

- When a patient is referred by a doctor or other professional person, the instructions given at the time of referral must be scrupulously carried out and not added to in any way.
- A patient should not be accepted for treatment if being treated by anyone else currently for the same or associated condition.
- When you accept a patient you are obligated to give the best treatment of which you are capable irrespective of race, creed or social status.

Towel draping

With every therapy treatment requiring the removal of some or most of a client's clothing, towel draping is an important aspect of a professional treatment. High standards in this area are an essential part of the professional image a therapist should adopt.

Therapists working in the field of massage and aromatherapy, for example, should possess a minimum of two large bath sheets per client and several hand towels. If a client is prone to feeling the cold, additional towels will be necessary.

256

There are several reasons for towel draping:

- It protects the modesty of the client.
- It reassures the client that the therapy is non-invasive even with the removal of clothing.
- It allows the body to remain warm. Correct room temperature should be approximately 75°F, but body temperature will always drop when a person is lying partly unclothed and in a horizontal position.
- It helps the client to relax. Always try to warm the towels beforehand.
- A good technique allows the therapist to work free from the encumbrance of towels or clothes whilst keeping the client warm.
- Good towel draping is part of a professional treatment.

By adopting the above principles, the therapist ensures the trust of his or her client.

Choice of towels

When choosing towels, although this is entirely the therapist's decision, the following points should be considered:

- Towelling sets should be kept to one colour and not patterned.
- Coloured towels should be matching or tone in with the couch linen.
- If you do not want white towels, warm pastel shades are preferable.
- Do not buy cheap towels as they may not hold the warmth and after several washes may become hard and rough.
- Make sure towels are of adequate length and width, as clients vary in height and size.
- Soak new towels in cold water before using for the first time to ensure the deep pile of the towel is retained.

Working with towels

When correct towel draping is adopted, any embarrassment to the therapist and client is alleviated. Only the area being worked on should be uncovered at any one time. This procedure ensures professional and ethical practice and demonstrates the standards of the therapist.

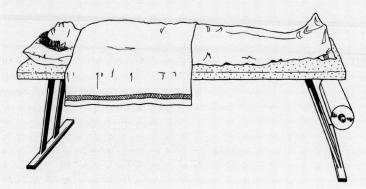

Towel draping starts when a client first approaches the couch and is helped on. Standards should be upheld throughout the treatment until you finally help the client to a sitting position and assist him or her off the couch.

Throughout every treatment, draping should always be neat and tidy, with towels being folded rather than rolled or bunched up. If towels are scrunched up, they inhibit you from working safely and correctly.

There are several good methods of towel draping taught. It becomes very easy to perform with continued practice and is effective. It should become a matter of course with every treatment given.

The therapy itself is not a complete treatment. The therapist should work holistically, and towel draping is part of an holistic treatment.

If the couch being used is portable, safety measures should be considered when helping the client on and off the couch:

- Hold the couch and allow the client to get on the opposite side. (Provide a step if necessary).
- When the client is ready to leave the couch, you can sit on the couch to stabilise it and help the client off the same side.

Remember, that as a therapist working with the public, you not only represent yourself but also the examining body with which you are qualified and the association of which you are a member. As professionals, therapists are always in a position of trust.

Contributed by Jane Evans

Patient support

The very quest for knowledge, which improves skill and efficiency, can easily obscure the biggest single ingredient of success – the patient. However luxurious your clinic, however excellent your treatments and however superb the products you use, they are of no avail if you neglect the opportunity to demonstrate them to the patients.

Patients should take precedence over all other considerations although the other factors may be valuable contributory ones.

Patients usually need understanding, frequently need sympathy and often need convincing that the treatment chosen for them is the right one. Very obviously, if the therapist is able to gain the co-operation of the patient, the treatment is likely to be more successful. There is no golden pathway to success in establishing the right relationship and confidence because so much depends on the personalities involved. There are however three considerations which it might be helpful to bear in mind:

- *The treatment should be such as to be and appear reasonable and the patient should benefit from it.* It may be necessary to explain in simple terms to patients the nature of the conditions for which they are being treated, followed by a brief description of the treatment they are to receive and its possible or expected results. It is acceptable to quote to the patient results which have been achieved in similar circumstances – but be careful not to overstate a case or create false optimism in the patient. From the patient's point of view the treatment should appear to be reasonable and an understanding of exactly what is involved should provide him or her with confidence and hopes of success in his or her case.

- *As far as possible the patient should enjoy the treatment.* This does not necessarily mean that the treatment will be without some discomfort or pain, but rather that the environment and attitudes should contribute to the greatest degree of comfort and peace of mind possible in the circumstances. The couch should be prepared before the patient arrives, and all materials likely to be required during the treatment should be ready. There should be a quiet air of efficiency and absence of rush and bustle and, as far as is possible, freedom from the interference of telephones or other interruptions. You should anticipate, as far as possible, the needs of the patient and do anything that will save him or her from embarrassment.

  Patients should be instructed clearly as to how much of their clothing it is necessary to remove, and the position of the changing room and toilet clearly indicated. When the patient is ready for treatment, he or she should be assisted on to the couch or treatment chair. Make sure that the patient is lying or sitting in a comfortable position. If the patient has a cold, place a supply of tissues alongside the couch. Should the patient wish to talk make a sincere effort to join in the conversation, but if the patient wishes to be quiet then respect this. Under no circumstances should the therapist impose his or her own problems on the patient.

- *The therapist should appear to be personally involved in the patient's progress.* A regular weighing and measuring of the patient, done personally by the therapist, helps to elicit a reciprocal responsibility from the patient. When the course of treatment is finished make it clear to the patient that you would like him or her to report in one or two weeks' time to be reweighed or remeasured or for such other checks as you may think necessary to enable you to keep an eye on his or her progress. If the patient does not present him or herself for this check there is no harm in sending a reminder card or letter similar to the ones that are often used by dentists.

An experienced therapist learns by touch, by speech and perhaps most of all by being a good listener, how to establish a good relationship with the patient and in this way accelerate the healing process.

Conclusion

Most of this book has been devoted to the knowledge of 'why' and 'how' on the basis that when the rationale is understood the decision of 'when, where and how much' is very much easier.

It is important to acquire knowledge and achieve still more expertise but it is even more important that these attributes should be directed by the belief in our own ability to contribute to the relief of pain, the reduction of disease and the restoration of health. The poet, Henry Twells, wrote:

'Your touch has still its ancient power, no word from you may fruitless fall, hear in this quiet evening hour and in your mercy heal us all.'

This is outside race and creed, beyond sectarianism or political convenience, it is personal dedication to a profession or part of a profession which, from time immemorial, has been dedicated to the service of its fellows, that by your treatment you enable people to face up to life with renewed energy, to regain health or rediscover the joy of living. This is the true reward of the physical therapist.

Some Useful Addresses

Examining bodies

Examining bodies who have separate Therapy examinations or a Therapy content in their general examinations:

City and Guilds of London Institute, 76 Portland Place, London W1N 4AA

Confederation of Beauty Therapy and Cosmetology, Parabola House, Parabola Road, Cheltenham, Glos. GL50 3AH
Tel: 01242 570284

ITEC (International Therapy Examination Council), 10/11 Heathfield Terrace, Chiswick, London W4 4JE

Professional organisations

Professional organisations offering their members services which include public indemnity insurance:

British Association of Beauty Therapy and Cosmetology, Parabola House, Parabola Road, Cheltenham, Glos. GL50 3AH
Tel: 01242 570284

Independent Professional Therapists' International, 8 Ordsall Road, Retford, Notts
Tel: 01777 700383, Fax: 01777 860374

Guild of Complementary Practitioners, Liddell House, Liddell Close, Finchampstead, Berkshire RG40 4NS
(General Secretary: John W. Beney)
Tel: 01189 735757, Fax: 01189 735767

Fellowship of Sports Masseurs and Therapists, B.M. Soigneur, London WC1N 3XX

Equipment suppliers

Ellisons Ltd, Crondal Road, Exhall, Coventry CV7 9NH
Tel: 01203 361619, Fax: 01203 644010

Carlton Professional, Carlton House, Commerce Way, Lancing, West Sussex BN15 8TA
Tel: 01903 761100, Fax: 01903 751111

Suppliers of essential oils and aromatherapy products

J.M.R. Paramedical Products (Yorkshire), 105 Otley Road, Harrogate, Yorkshire HG2 0AG
Tel: 01423 505707

Teaching aids ITEC Teachers Training Diploma Course details from:
ITEC, James House, Oakelbrook Mill, Newent, Glos. GL18 1HD
Tel: 01531 821875, Fax: 01531 822425

Electro-epilation: A *practical approach for* NVQ *level* 3 by Elizabeth Cartwright,
Gill Morris and Michelle Sullivan, published by Stanley Thornes
(1995).

Modular teaching systems available from:

Kajpak Publications, Barncroft, Pinfold Hill, Curbar, Nr Sheffield,
Yorks
Tel/Fax: 01433 630437 or 01335 370904

and from Elizabeth Cartwright Ltd, East Midlands College,
Halliday House, 2 Wilson Street, Derby DE1 1PG
Tel: 01332 205788, Fax: 01332 205783

Nutrition advisers training courses:

Paul Godwin, BA, DC, Cert.Ed., Lauriston House, London Road,
Basingstoke RG21 4AA
Tel/Fax: 01256 475728

Index